Success is best measured by how far you've come
with the talents you've been given.

Anonymous

This book is dedicated to my mother, Mary Lou Sullivan. Her legacy is the fact that she raised six children to be upstanding, contributing members of their communities. She worked hard, always with pride in what she did, and contributed to the lives of many people. She made a difference with her life. I hope I can say the same when my time comes.

My mom left my life too early, just prior to her retirement, at age 61. She practiced a healthy lifestyle and should have lived a long life. Instead she died on 10/20/97 as the result of a traumatic brain injury, caused by a fall on stairs in her home. She was never able to do all the things she said she'd do "someday." Her death, more than my own brain injury, pushes me to try to make a difference for other brain injury survivors, to work to increase awareness of this "silent epidemic," to get the word out about the importance of preventing traumatic brain injuries and to advocate within the health care system and the community for persons with disabilities.

Contents

Foreword

If you are coping with a brain injury — either personally, within your family, or among your friends — you have just opened the right book.

The Brain Injury Survival Kit is unique in the world of self-help literature. It isn't written by just another doctor who likes to write, or by a brain injury survivor who likes to share, it is a combination of the two — and you are the beneficiary.

Cheryle Sullivan, MD, knows brain injury — BI — and she knows it intimately. Before her own accidents, she dealt with BI in her immediate family, so the road has been long and hard, but instructive. As a physician, she thinks scientifically, making the kind of connections between neurology and everyday reality that escape most of her peers, and virtually all of ours. She has walked the walk and now she is talking the talk — to you.

The *Survival Kit* is a practical approach to living every day (every single day, since it provides 365 tips, tools and tricks…) with a brain injury. The severity of the impairment will, of course, dictate the utility of what you learn, but there is clearly something for everybody in this great collection of helpful hints.

Those of us in the field of education, prevention, and treatment understand that, historically, brain injury has been a hidden epidemic, plaguing the world for centuries, without its due notice. Unless a head injury resulted in obvious surgery, facial alteration, or physical impairment, most brain dysfunctions were invisible to others. Injuries resulting from falls at home or collisions on the football field had been dismissed as mere "concussions," where the survivor was merely "knocked out."

No more. Between America's professional sports and the mid-East wars of the new century, awareness has risen. People are beginning to wear helmets when skiing, riding bicycles or playing on skateboards. Schools and teams are collecting baseline data for annual comparisons to monitor the status of basic brain functions. Emergency rooms are doing follow-ups on the most minor of head injuries. Intensive Care Units and Rehab centers are saving lives and brain function with new drugs, machines, and techniques.

Knowing about all of this progress, Dr. Sullivan has stepped forward to serve the cause. I first met her at a Brain Injury 101 class that she was teaching in Colorado Springs, at Penrose Hospital, where I served as Director of Rehabilitation Services. I was (and am) President of the Board of Directors of the Brain Injury Association of Colorado (BIAC), whose mission is to enhance the quality of life for survivors of brain injury and their families, and BI 101 is one of our community classes.

Beyond her vast knowledge of the neurological basics of BI, I was struck by Dr. Sullivan's common-sense approach to daily life, and, of course, her vibrant sense of humor. She was amazingly direct and transparent about her own impairments, often laughing at herself when a word escaped immediate recall; she would calmly capture the moment and use it as an example of impaired brain function. Such spontaneous honesty made her more human and approachable to the audience — many of whom were also survivors.

Increased awareness and advanced technology have created the greatest population of known brain injury survivors in the history of the world, so Dr. Sullivan's book is a timely and valuable contribution. If you are living with or near brain injury you will immediately recognize the physical, mental and emotional challenges cited in this book, and you will appreciate the experience-based solutions offered. I am proud to recommend it.

Gary A. Morse, MA, MS
Vice President, Human Resources,
Penrose-St. Francis Health Services,
Colorado Springs, CO

Preface

It is hard for me to believe that it has been 10 years since my mom's death from a Traumatic Brain Injury (TBI) and 5 years since the TBI that changed the course of my own life.

I was one of the 20% of mild traumatic brain injury (MTBI) survivors who were fortunate to receive cognitive rehabilitation services. Through work with two cognitive therapists, several neuropsychologists, and my physical medicine and rehabilitation physician, I was able to maximize the use of cognitive "orthoses." I also had the benefit of my past experience as a family physician, physician manager, and general aviation pilot. In these activities, I had learned to use many tools and strategies to maximize my abilities to deal with the ordinary, as well as the unexpected.

Many other conditions exhibit cognitive problems similar to those resulting from TBI, including brain injuries from other than traumatic causes, learning disabilities, developmental disabilities, stress, and the aging process. Many people living with cognitive challenges don't have the benefit of having developed the skills necessary for coping and overcoming these obstacles. One of my goals, in *Brain Injury Survival Kit*, is to provide those who have had brain injuries and those with cognitive function loss due to other factors with some new tools and strategies to help deal with the mental challenges they face every day. This information will relate to memory, time management, organization, as well as other areas that effect cognitive function. In addition to dealing with specific tools and strategies, I will cover some general health issues that impact cognitive function, including illness, stress, exercise, diet, relaxation, and sleep. How we take care of our general health has a great impact on how well we function cognitively.

The ultimate goal of *Brain Injury Survival Kit* is to have all readers—those living with brain injuries and those living or working with someone who is dealing with cognitive problems—gain from it some readily usable strategies to maximize their cognitive abilities.

Do not wait; the time will never be "just right."
Start where you stand, and work with whatever
tools you may have at your command, and better
tools will be found as you go along.

Napoleon Hill

Acknowledgments

Great things are done by a series of small things brought together.

Vincent van Gogh

To Denise Kiepe, RN, Senior Care Coordinator at the Longmont Kaiser Permanente Facility, who was there for me when things were too much for me to handle. To Julie Stapleton, MD, one of the most caring and compassionate doctors I've ever met. She really "gets it" about the way it is for those of us dealing with MTBI, and goes above and beyond what a typical doctor does for her patients. She is a real advocate. To the Mapleton Rehabilitation Center team who supported and guided me along a path I didn't always want to take, to a place where I could then take up the journey on my own again. To Don Gerber, PhD of Craig Hospital, who listened, helped problem-solve, gave of himself and his time, and really cared.

To my dad, who put up with my lack of memory and navigating ability during our trip to Ireland without complaint. You were a great tour guide. I hope this book will offer you tips to help you deal with the consequences of your own 2005 TBI. To Earl and Henrietta Tilford, friends who were there for the long haul, for all the transportation help I needed, as well as moral support. They taught me the importance of accepting help when offered, and more so, of asking for help when I needed it. To Bethel Barger, who invited me to her home for weekly knitting sessions. You taught me to knit and shared the wisdom and common sense of your 90+ years of healthy living. To Joel Kiester, who took me flying when I couldn't fly myself and kept my spirits up. To Melanie Shaha, who gave time she didn't have to spare to edit my writing. To the Brain Injury Association of Colorado, and specifically Peggy and Theodora, for supporting my need to spread the word about TBI.

Last, to all the brain injury survivors who have offered me support as well as information, transportation, and companionship. It is so much easier to talk to someone who really knows what dealing with brain injury is all about.

Life breaks everyone, but some people become stronger in the broken places.

Ernest Hemingway

Brain Injury Survival Kit

CHAPTER 1

Put Your House In Order: Strive for a Healthier Lifestyle

What is important is not what happens to us,
but how we respond to what happens to us.
                                    Jean-Paul Sartre

All of us, those with brain injuries or not, know how hard it is to concentrate and think when we are tired, hungry, upset, or distracted. To maximize our cognitive abilities (the way we think, understand, and process information), we have to take care of ourselves, both physically and emotionally. Throughout my career as a family physician, I actively spoke on health-related issues, in my exam rooms and in my community. When I spoke on almost any subject, such as preventing heart disease, staying healthy during cold and flu season, or dealing with menopause issues, I always talked about the basic foundations of health. No matter what specific topic I was discussing, I always spoke of certain common elements. These are: diet, exercise, rest, and stress reduction.

These concepts run throughout every aspect of our health. We cannot always control what happens to us, but we can make our bodies as healthy as possible to better withstand physical and emotional stresses placed on them. These same elements are vitally important in successfully dealing with the consequences of brain injury.

Diet

I have heard or read the expression many times: "You are what you eat." Besides leading to premature health problems, a poor diet can lessen our ability to handle stress. Here are some basics that I have found of benefit over the years, and especially more recently when dealing with the after-effects of my own traumatic brain injury (TBI):

♦ **Don't skip meals.** Skipping meals can lead to *hypoglycemia*, or low blood sugar. People who have hypoglycemia feel sluggish and lack energy. Many studies over the years have shown that school children perform much better when starting their day with breakfast. You cannot run a car without gas, and it is hard for your brain, as well as your body, to run well without food for fuel.

♦ **"Graze,"** especially when stressed, exercising, or trying to accomplish more than usual. Grazing is eating more frequent, smaller amounts throughout the day. By taking breaks to eat snacks or small meals, an added plus is that you give yourself needed rests from continued cognitive activity.

— When performing physical activity, make sure to take along and eat healthy snacks. This helps keep energy up and prevents fatigue, which tends to worsen cognitive function. Snacks to take along include nuts, dried fruit, granola, or energy bars and, of course, something to drink.

— Always pack a granola bar or two and a bottle of water in your backpack when away from home, as well as have some stashed in your vehicle.

♦ Garbage in, garbage out. I have heard this expression used in many ways, but I know it applies to our diets. If we spend every day eating potato chips and French fries, and drinking soda, we cannot expect our bodies and brains to perform very well. I believe an occasional excess, eating too much or the "wrong" things, is not a big deal. But, we need to consider what we eat day in and day out and work toward a goal of eating in a healthier fashion.

What Is a "Healthy Diet?"

Many healthy—and some not so healthy—diet recommendations are made by all kinds of "experts," real or not. I will only tell you what seems important to me, and what I try to follow:

♦ Eat reasonable amounts. The answer to maintaining a reasonable body weight is to eat the amount of calories your body burns or, if you want to eat more, burn more calories with exercise and activity. Skipping meals actually slows your metabolism, as the body goes into a "conserve" mode when it does not see enough fuel in the system.

♦ Measure your food. One of the best ways to eat the right amounts of food is to actually measure your portions. Most recipes and packages of food tell you how many they serve, and what amount is a portion size. If a dish says it serves four people, divide it into four portions and, if eating alone, freeze the extras for meals at later dates. If something says a half-cup is a serving, measure it out. You will be amazed at how much (or little) this actually is, compared to how much you usually serve yourself.

♦ Eat at the right times. We need to eat when our body needs the energy, so the calories are burned rather than being stored. We then will also have enough fuel in our system throughout the day to prevent hypoglycemia. For me, especially since my last TBI, I am the most active physically and cognitively in the morning. I am often physically active in the afternoons, although with less cognitive activity. In the evenings, I am usually neither physically nor cognitively active. That means I need the most fuel in the morning, less in the afternoon, and the least in the evenings. This is very different from most people's dietary habits, when they skip breakfast, eat a light lunch or none at all, and eat a large supper, often later in the evening.

— Even if you do not have the time or inclination to eat a large breakfast, moving more calories to earlier in the day by increasing what you eat for breakfast or adding a mid-morning snack at the expense of a large supper will be beneficial.

— Taking away some of your supper calories and adding a mid-afternoon snack also helps.

♦ Eat the right kinds of food. This is where things get controversial, especially when talking about weight loss. There are diets promoting every type of eating, from high-protein, low-carbohydrate, all-grapefruit, low-protein, and on and on. Similar diet programs seem to surface over the years, with new names attached. I am not going to discuss the pros and cons of these different diets, but will give you some basics that I try to follow.

— Limit meat intake. Many studies over the years have shown a link between diets high in meat and cancers, especially colon and breast cancers. I try to limit my meat intake, and I try to eat mostly poultry and leaner cuts of red meat.

— Measure portions. Meat consumption is another area where measuring portions helps you be aware of how much you should eat. A good tip is that a meat serving is about the size of a deck of cards, or the palm of an adult's hand.

— Preparation makes a difference. A serving of broiled, boiled, or grilled meat has less fat than the same serving deep-fried, fried, or baked in the meat's own juices.

♦ Eat more fresh fruits and vegetables, as these have been show to help lower our cancer risk. They are also rich in antioxidants, nutrients that protect our brains and bodies from free radicals, the unstable molecules that are thought to diminish brain function and overall health. Fruits and vegetables also make good grazing foods although, as with everything else, portion size is important. Too much of a good thing is still too much, as far as calories and weight gain are concerned. Fried okra, zucchini, French fries, or onion rings do not have the same health benefits as the same vegetables raw, or an orange, or a handful of blueberries. And it is much better to eat fresh fruit than to drink fruit juice. The juice has more concentrated sugar and less fiber than the fruit and for many does not seem as filling. With juices, it is also easy to exceed portion sizes. This is especially true when a bottle contains two to two-and-a-half servings but can be easily finished in one sitting. Read the juice bottle label to see how many servings it contains.

♦ Eat foods high in fiber. Not only is fiber filling, helping you limit overeating and maintain a reasonable weight, it also helps regulate your bowel and manage conditions such as constipation and irritable bowel syndrome. When eaten regularly as part of a diet low in saturated fat and cholesterol, soluble fiber has been shown to help lower your cholesterol and may also help reduce the risk of diseases like diabetes and colon and rectal cancer. Because of eating so many processed foods, Americans tend to get much less than the recommended amounts of fiber in their diet.

♦ Eat fish. Research shows that eating oily fish containing omega-3 fatty acids is linked to better health, particularly lowering your risk of death from coronary artery disease. These fatty acids are concentrated in the brain and are associated with cognitive function. Omega-3 oils may also be of benefit in preventing some of the effects of brain injury. These fats count as "healthy" fats, protecting against high cholesterol and inflammation in our bodies. Sources of omega-3 include cold-water fish (for example, salmon, trout, tuna, halibut, mackerel, and herring), flaxseed and flaxseed oil, and walnuts and walnut oil.

Supplements

As with many medical conditions, much is made of dietary supplements for helping memory and other cognitive issues after brain injury. The U.S. Food and Drug Administration (FDA) does not regulate these supplements. The dietary supplement manufacturer is responsible for ensuring that a dietary supplement is safe before it is marketed. The FDA is responsible for taking action against any unsafe dietary supplement product after it reaches the market. Generally, manufacturers do not need to register their products with the FDA nor get FDA approval before producing or selling dietary supplements. Manufacturers must make sure that product label information is truthful and not misleading. Many are sold based on personal testimonials to their effectiveness rather than any evidence from scientific studies. They usually have statements on their labels saying they can make no claim to have medical benefits. Please consult with your medical team before taking any of these. Nutrients work best when they're consumed in the foods we eat, so try to eat a well-balanced, healthy diet.

♦ Take your vitamins. Do consider adding a good multivitamin/mineral supplement to your daily regimen. The best multivitamins for memory should include 100% of the recommended daily allowance of vitamins B6, B12, and folic acid, as well as zinc and boron. The B vitamins, especially B6, B12, and folic acid, protect the brain by breaking down homocysteine, an amino acid that is toxic to nerve cells. They also are involved in manufacturing the red blood cells that carry oxygen. The best sources for these nutrients are dark-colored, leafy greens such as spinach, and broccoli, asparagus, strawberries, melons, black beans, soybeans, and other legumes and citrus fruits.

♦ Get more antioxidants. Vitamins E and C and beta carotene, all known antioxidants, help fight off free radicals. Free radicals are by-products of normal oxygen use by our body's cells, and they are linked to disease and aging. Antioxidants also improve the flow of oxygen through the body and brain. Scientific data suggest that antioxidants help retard the aging process, maintaining memory function in the process. Sources of these antioxidants include blueberries and other berries, sweet potatoes, beets, red tomatoes, spinach, broccoli, green tea, nuts and seeds, citrus fruits, and liver.

♦ Limit caffeine intake. A little may perk you up, but too much can be distracting. Caffeine is contained in many energy supplements and drinks, as well as in coffee, tea, cocoa, and chocolate.

Exercise

As a family physician interacting with my patients, I often recommended some type of regular exercise as part of the treatment for many health concerns. The many benefits of exercise include managing weight, helping with stress and insomnia, treating and preventing arthritis and other musculoskeletal problems, improving the odds of preventing cancers, and increasing the possibility of living longer and with better maintained physical and mental functioning. Research has shown that exercise aids in the recovery of people who have had brain injuries. What types of exercise are best?

♦ Mix it up. Most of us are best served with a mix of aerobic exercises (brisk exercise that makes your heart and lungs work harder) and weight training. Aerobic exercise increases circulation—the flow of blood and oxygen to the brain—and helps us perform better mentally. It also increases our metabolism, helping to control weight, which lowers the risk of developing diseases that worsen brain function. Weight training helps with balance, endurance, and muscle strength.

♦ **Pick an exercise routine you enjoy.** If you hate what you are doing, you will have a hard time maintaining the program. Healthy diet and exercise regimens should be considered life-long practices, as the benefits of both are quickly lost if not continued.

♦ **Stretch.** Stretching maintains joint flexibility and helps prevent injuries while exercising. The best exercise routine is to: stretch, warm-up, exercise, cool-down, and stretch again. Warm-up and cool-down periods involve a few minutes of doing a particular exercise activity at a slower pace, or by taking a slow walk before and after playing a game of tennis, golf, or another activity. Warm-up periods allow your muscles to warm up, so that they are less likely to tear with excessive stretching during the exercise activity. After activity, the cool-down allows fatigued muscles a chance to recover. The stretching before and after are also very important to prevent injuries. Maintaining joint flexibility is important in maintaining and protecting joint function. You can learn stretching routines from books, online web sites, at health and fitness clubs, and from your health care professionals.

♦ **Join up.** Many people find it easier to exercise consistently if they do it with a friend or take a class. You can swim, do water aerobics, walk, jog, bike (please wear a helmet), dance, or choose from many other activities. Many can be done with little or no equipment or cost, and can be done from home or while traveling. For seniors or those with health problems, many community recreation centers offer programs specifically tailored to your needs (such as the Silver Sneakers Program in my community). Chair-based programs (in which the exercises are performed while seated) are available on videos or DVDs.

♦ **Write it down.** Keeping a log or diary of exercise goals and actual practices helps maintain a consistent routine. Set a goal to exercise most days of the week, usually planning to miss one or two days at the most. Each day, write what you did and, if you missed unexpectedly, why you missed, so that you justify to yourself that you had a good reason.

♦ **Count your steps.** Wear a pedometer, so you have an idea how active—or sedentary—you are throughout each day. By monitoring your steps during the day, you can see if you need to pick it up as the day progresses to get to your minimum goal. (The American Heart Association goal is 10,000 steps a day.)

♦ **Walk more.** To increase your steps in a day, simple things like parking farther away at a store, using a portable telephone in your home, walking in the house while talking, and getting rid of the TV remote control and getting up to change channels all contribute to more activity.

♦ **Lift weights.** Weight training can be as easy as lifting a can of soup or using stretchy bands or basic weights bought at any sporting goods or general merchandise store. You can find recommendations for weight-based exercise programs in books, online, or from your health professional. Some simple weight-training routines can help maintain your ability to climb stairs safely, get up out of a chair, carry and put away groceries, and even better maintain your balance to avoid falls. Again, as with aerobic activity, start low and go slow. Increase the weight amount or the number of repetitions no more often than weekly and usually only one or the other in a week, not both. We want to see fast results when we start an exercise program, but when it comes to weight training, being a tortoise rather than a hare helps prevent injuries that could make us stop exercising.

Rest

Many people do not get enough sleep. This can lessen our ability to handle stress and make us function less productively and accurately. People who have had brain injuries often need even more sleep than those without brain injuries—as much as 10+ hours a night. This is especially true in the early post-injury period. We may also need frequent breaks or naps throughout the day. Your brain needs to rest in order to heal.

♦ **Schedule sleep and rest.** Set up a regular sleep and rest schedule. Allow plenty of time to sleep, as well as rest breaks during the day. The goal is to rest before you are overly tired. When you use up your energy reserves, you often cannot restore them with one night of good sleep—it may take days to restore them.

♦ Take your time. Don't rush back to daily activities, such as work or school. Consider returning for part of a day, maybe a few days scattered over the week. If you do not start a day as fresh as the day before, you likely did too much the previous day and are not ready to increase your activity level.

Stress Reduction

Stress is certainly not limited to those of us dealing with a TBI, nor to our families. Stress was a common complaint among my patients over the years. There are all sorts of methods recommended for stress management; pick what works for you and what you feel you can do and practice it. If you have a stress management tool, but never practice using it, when you are stressed, it is not likely to work very well for you.

◆ **Breathe.** In addition to providing the needed oxygen to the brain, taking a deep breath is relaxing, and many forms of yoga and meditation involve learning how to breathe to help with improved physical and mental function.

◆ **Do yoga.** Yoga helps with physical functioning by improving strength, flexibility, balance, and coordination. It also helps with emotional functioning by contributing to improved relaxation, sleep, and mental functioning. Yoga can be learned and practiced individually, using books, video tapes, and CDs available for instruction, or by taking a class.

◆ **Love your pet.** I would not recommend bringing a new pet into the home while trying to deal with the consequences of a recent brain injury, because you are likely to be overwhelmed already with your normal responsibilities. If you already have a pet, however, the process of caring for your pet can be relaxing and stress-reducing. Your pet also provides companionship, which is important when you often feel socially isolated by your brain injury. Walking your dog, providing for your pet's needs, and playing with and petting them are all things that help you stay grounded and relaxed.

♦ **Get a hobby.** I found that, after my TBI, with the extra time needed for sleep and the inefficiency and distractibility caused by my cognitive deficits, I would attempt to spend all of my waking hours doing productive work, trying to "accomplish things" each day. This was at the expense of those activities that were most beneficial to my health: exercise, eating, rest, and fun. I did not make time for hobbies early on. In addition to being fun, hobbies are stress-reducers and, in learning new things, we promote improved cognitive function and healthier living habits.

♦ **Sign up social support.** Having family support or a strong social network is important for good health, including reducing stress. It has also been shown to help people recover from cancer, and it is a factor in how well people recover from TBIs. In addition to providing needed care and services, your family and friends provide encouragement and can be partners in exercise and fun activities.

♦ **Join a support group.** According to scientific studies, women do better after breast cancer when they participate in support groups. Similar benefits are seen with other conditions. Brain injury support groups, accessed through your state Brain Injury Association offices, offer access to other people who are dealing with the same issues after brain injuries. In these groups, you can network with others who are living with brain injury, as well as with their family members.

♦ **Find spiritual support.** Research has shown that you generally have a healthier lifestyle if you include religion or spirituality. For many, prayer is a stress reliever. For those uncomfortable with prayer, meditation is an alternative.

♦ **Keep a positive attitude.** Our attitude has a great effect on how we deal with things, good and bad. It is one of the known factors affecting outcome after TBI. Depending on our point of view, something can be stressful or a challenge. We need to find ways to eliminate negative thought patterns and take on more positive, affirming thought patterns.

Most of the important things in the world have been accomplished by people who have kept on trying when there seemed to be no hope at all.
                                            Dale Carnegie

CHAPTER 2

The Game Plan

Believing in our hearts that who we are is enough
is the key to a more satisfying and balanced life.
                                                    Ellen Sue Stern

A brain injury is not something a person can out-muscle. Although I have succeeded in almost every goal I have ever set by working hard, trying hard to remember something or to pay attention and concentrate after a brain injury seldom works. You cannot work hard to see again if you are blind, or to hear again if you are deaf. Especially in the early weeks and months after my brain injury, this "work-hard mentality" led me to feel frustrated and discouraged. Working hard using those methods that succeeded for me in the past did not get the results I wanted and needed. This can lead to a feeling of being overwhelmed, confused, and even more fatigued. However, trying hard to learn to use new effective strategies and tools for retrieving information or successfully accomplishing tasks does help. Cognitive therapy focuses on regaining those skills we have lost as well as learning to use tools and strategies to compensate for abilities that have been permanently changed because of brain injury. It is much like physical therapy, in which a person who has lost a leg does not expect to get that leg back, but to learn to use tools and strategies to compensate for the loss of the leg. By using these new tools and strategies to manage the cognitive losses due to brain injury, we are working smarter rather than working harder.

♦ Set your goals. You must realign your goals and attitudes related to how you function. A friend from my brain injury support group expressed it in a way that I like. He said that excellence is not the same thing as perfection, and that the goal should be to strive for excellence, not perfection. Perfection is a nearly impossible goal for everyone, those with a brain injury or not. A few other "truisms" that must be realigned include:

— If you can't do it right, don't do it at all. If we treated this as fact we would never try anything, as you rarely do things right as you are learning them. You likely did not ride a bike for the first time without falling, nor hit a baseball the first time you swung at one. Most people with brain injuries can learn new things, but they may take longer to do it. If we and the people around us have patience and give us support, we can usually learn how to do something new, often using the tools and strategies we have learned to compensate for our memory issues.

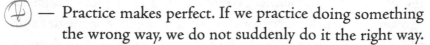

— Practice makes perfect. If we practice doing something the wrong way, we do not suddenly do it the right way.

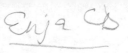

Instead, we should say "Practice perfect makes perfect." Practicing doing something the correct way, even if doing it more slowly and deliberately, will help us learn to do it the right way.

— If it was important, you would have remembered it. I have heard this from many people, and, in fact, I used to say this when I forgot things in the past. This is certainly not true. We can compare our short-term memory to the clipboard on a computer. When you "cut" something, if you "cut" something else before you paste the original material, it is lost. In your computer, you can return to the original document to retrieve it, but in your memory, there is no original document. If a piece of new information is lost from your short-term memory, it never made it into your long-term memory, so it is not there to retrieve. I know some people think we are not trying hard enough when we cannot remember something they ask us about. If that piece of information didn't make it into longer-term memory, it is not retrievable, no matter how hard we try. We can frustrate ourselves trying to find something that is not there, or we can move on. We likely will not be able to "fix" our short-term memory issue, but we can successfully get around it using strategies and tools.

Typical of those of us who have sustained a brain injury, as well as of our families and supporters, I repeatedly asked members of my rehabilitation team "When will I be better? When will I be 'back to normal?' and When can I go back to my job?"

As I learned over time, recovery takes time and is a difficult journey for most who undertake it.

Also, "normal" must take on a new definition. When someone loses a leg, no one expects that person to "get back to normal." The expectation is for that person to learn to compensate with a new prosthesis. Because brain injury is invisible to many, the expectation is that the person will return to his previous self. This is often not the case.

I was told early on that a brain injury was different from many other types of injuries, in that it left those who live with its effects with an "altered sense of self." The very person you were is changed: how you think, how you feel emotionally, how you interact socially. In our recovery, we not only need to rebuild our cognitive abilities through learning new tools and strategies, we need to rebuild our sense of self. We need to become comfortable with the new person we have become. I don't know where this quotation originated, but I heard it at a rally prior to our annual Pikes Peak Challenge fund-raiser in Colorado, and I think it really speaks to this: We are not who we were, be who we are.

The problem is that we, our support people, and our therapists, get so wrapped up in finding answers for the physical and cognitive symptoms of brain injury—pain, fatigue, memory problems, and more—that we tend to overlook the emotional devastation that has occurred. As frustrated as I was by my difficulties with memory, fatigue, attention, vision, and more, I was more bothered by the changes in my life caused by those difficulties. I did not find peace when I learned to use tools and strategies to compensate for many of my cognitive deficits. Instead, I pushed myself to work longer and longer, taking on more and more projects, trying to return to the highly productive person I had been in the past. I found peace only when I eventually realized that I could still contribute and be of value, but in different ways from that highly productive person I had been. I found new ways to enjoy life. I gave up a lifetime of playing softball as well as skiing and all the friends I had with those activities. I've moved into camping and traveling, expanded my aviation interests, and have an entirely new circle of friends to share these activities with.

♦ You are not what you "do." We are human "beings" not human "doings." It is healthier to identify myself as a woman who practiced medicine and flew an airplane, not as a doctor and a pilot. When we lose the ability to "do" things we used to do before our brain injury, we feel like we have lost who we were. We have lost what we did, but we still are people with a lot of abilities to offer to our families, friends, and communities. This is similar to the concept in disability awareness of using "people first" language. We are not brain injured; we are persons with a brain injury. We are not our medical diagnosis, any more than we are the job we do, the make of car we drive, the brand of clothing we wear, or the type of food we eat.

The following chapters contain specific tips, tools, and strategies to deal with the cognitive issues related to impaired brain functioning. Some of these you will already be using and others will not fit your needs.

Take what you can use, adapt and adjust it to fit you, and find the best set of tips, tools, and strategies to make your day-to-day functioning easier and better. You might consider starting with something easy to add to your routine, or something to help with a particular frustration in your life. I strongly recommend that you do not try to incorporate many of the new things you learn here all at once. That's a sure path to failure.

We have choices after a brain injury. We can chose to continue being frustrated by our inability to accomplish things because of distractions, forgetfulness, and other cognitive issues, or we can take on new strategies and tools to help us to function at the highest level we can. These new strategies, like taking on a new haircut or a new pair of glasses, in time become the "new" me, just as, throughout our lives, we have adapted and changed to fit the requirements of the world around us.

People with cognitive changes caused by aging have an advantage in my opinion. They have a gradual onset of symptoms, so that they can gradually adapt as needed to deal with these changes. With a brain injury, these changes occur instantaneously. We must suddenly let go of the old "me" and the way we did things in the past and take on a new "me," as well as the new strategies and tools needed to deal with that new person. We also have to learn to like and value the new "me."

It can be done. Many before us have succeeded, including many with severe cognitive deficits. How well we recover from our brain injuries depends on who we are: our attitudes, our work ethic, our ability to ask for and use help, and our ability to accept and even thrive on change. Our recovery is an ongoing process. We will at times have setbacks, need new strategies and tools to deal with changes in our lives, and have made available to us new technologies as they are developed. This is not a one-time fix situation. Prepare yourself for some work ahead.

applies to grieving as well!

I gain strength, courage, and confidence by every experience in which I must stop and look fear in the face. . . . I say to myself, I've lived through this and can take the next thing that comes along. . . . We must do things we think we cannot do.

Eleanor Roosevelt

CHAPTER 3

Energy

One of the things that has helped me as much as any other, is not how long I am going to live but how much I can do while living.
George Washington Carver

Fatigue is actually considered a physical, not a cognitive symptom, and it affects nearly everyone who has had a traumatic brain injury (TBI). It has been described as one of the most limiting consequences of brain injury. Nothing affects my cognitive ability more than fatigue. Managing your cognitive energy is one of the most important things you can do to help you perform at the highest level possible.

In the first days and weeks after my TBI, fatigue was an overwhelming problem. I wanted to sleep almost constantly, at the expense of any social or physical activities—even eating. I thought I knew what fatigue felt like after four years of medical school, three years of residency, and many years of being on call as a family physician. I didn't have a clue. This was a fatigue that was so deep, I had no choice but to drop what I was doing and rest or I would literally drop. I can remember falling asleep in my chair with my supper plate on my lap, on buses going to or from medical appointments, and even at my computer. It was as if someone turned out the lights.

Somewhere around the second month after my TBI, the general fatigue seemed to improve. I found I could work many hours in my yard without getting tired, but minimal cognitive activity—reading, working on my finances, even talking on the phone or attending a meeting—would wear me out and require a prolonged rest. I was doing some flying with an instructor, both to learn new things as well as to keep up an activity I loved. After one hour of flying, I would go home and sleep for two or three hours to recover. I also was very fatigued after dealing with any emotional issues, and early on after a brain injury there are plenty of those. When I began my outpatient neuro-trauma rehabilitation, I learned more about fatigue.

Basically, we face two kinds of fatigue: physical and mental. You can divide mental into cognitive (thinking) and emotional (feeling). We expend energy for physical, cognitive, and emotional functioning, and then we have reserve stores of energy. Figure 3.1 shows the typical person's energy distribution and that of a person who has had a mild TBI. Not only does the person with TBI use more energy than in the past to deal with physical, cognitive, and emotional activities, but his energy reserves are diminished. What I found, and many others have reported, is that when you deplete your energy reserves, it takes days to restore them. Overdoing it on a Monday or Tuesday resulted in me being excessively tired until the weekend, when I could spend an entire day sleeping. One good night's rest was

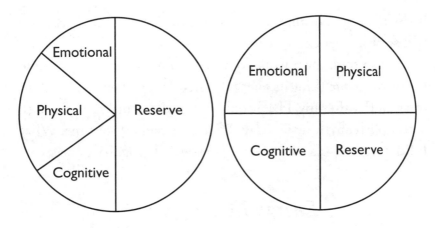

Figure 3.1: Energy Pie. Normal (left) and after a mild brain injury (right).

Copyright © Mary Lou Acimovic, MA.

not enough to restore my energy balance. I seem to start the day with less energy, use it up more rapidly than in the past and have trouble refreshing it with a good night's rest.

When fatigued, everything we do seems to take more effort. We also make mistakes and get frustrated. Early on, my typical reaction to being tired during the day was to "gut it out" and try to finish the task I had scheduled. Not only would it take me much longer to do when I was tired, but the quality of my work suffered.

My cognitive therapists as well as my social worker were constantly reminding me that, when I was tired, it was my brain telling me to slow down, and that the brain healed when I rested. Now, even more than five years after my TBI, I typically need nine to ten hours of sleep a night to feel adequately rested. I schedule a break during the day, and if the morning has been very "cognitive," this time is used for a nap. With a less cognitively demanding morning, a period of minimally cognitive activity will suffice to re-energize me.

It also took me a while to understand and accept that time is not the same thing as energy. When I was unable to work in the months after my TBI, I could not understand why I failed to accomplish anything in a day. After all, I had lots of time. What I did not have was a lot of energy, especially cognitive energy.

Explains a lot!

Energy Management

♦ Pace yourself. Consider the energy demands for the day due to expected physical, cognitive, and emotional activities.

♦ Rest when you are tired. Pushing on will lead to worsening function and the chance of a "meltdown."

♦ Take frequent breaks, especially before you are tired.

— General breaks. Stop for lunch, coffee, or go for a walk.

— Cognitive breaks. Go to a nonstimulating place to rest your brain. Avoid visual, auditory, or mental stimulation for a short period.

♦ Take naps. I find setting an alarm to prevent prolonged sleeping helps me feel rested, but doesn't interfere with my nighttime sleep.

♦ Sit. If energy is an issue, sit down as much as you can. Standing up uses a lot of energy. Put a stool in the kitchen, so that you can sit down to prepare food, stir things on the stove, and do other tasks.

♦ Plan your energy use. Look at your day and week and plan out your energy use.

— Don't just plan the number or hours of activities for a day, but plan based on the energy needs of those activities. A hair appointment demands a lot less cognitive energy than a meeting with a lawyer, insurance agent, or Social Security Administration staff member.

— Look at planned activities for the entire day or week when considering adding something else, as you may already be at your limit for that day or week.

♦ Plan for learning. Anticipate that, in new environments or when taking on new tasks, higher cognitive demands will be associated with "new learning" as opposed to your usual activities.

♦ Prevent overload. Pay attention to signs of fatigue and consider that they may be different from the warning signs of fatigue prior to your TBI. Some examples include:

— Less ability to follow conversations

— Slower speed of thinking

— More disorganized thinking

— Losing train of thought

— Increased errors

— Trouble finding words or substituting wrong words

— Dizziness

— Blurred vision

— Headache

♦ Use strategies and tools. Use the compensating strategies and tools provided by your rehabilitation team and in the later chapters of this book to lessen your daily cognitive demand.

— The more you use the strategies and tools, the more automatic they become and the less thought they require.

— The more you do automatically, without using a lot of brain energy, the more brain energy left for other things and the longer you can function cognitively in a day.

— For example, I don't waste my cognitive energy stores worrying about whether or not I'll remember an appointment because I enter all of them in my personal digital assistant (PDA) with reminders. Similarly, I don't spend a lot of energy looking for my keys, because they are put in a specific place in my home every time I come in.

♦ Say no. You must be willing to bail on a "bad brain day". If you wake up tired and are having difficulty thinking, seriously consider canceling planned activities. How much benefit will you get out of them anyway?

Safety Issues

If you have had a brain injury and have cognitive fatigue issues, be very aware of safety concerns. When I am tired, I know my brain is not functioning as well as is "normal" for me. My reaction time is slower, as is my processing of information. I also have a harder time paying attention, and my memory works less well. This is not the time for me to be driving a car or flying an airplane. When I have to drive into urban traffic to do a brain injury presentation, I usually plan to arrive at least 30 minutes early to allow for rest prior to my program. I also usually plan to rest before or on the way driving back home.

I have been blessed in that, after my TBI, I retained the insight and judgment to monitor myself, and not put myself and others in danger by attempting these activities when tired. Not everyone is as fortunate.

♦ Listen to your inner voice. If you have intact insight, listen to it. If not, you need to find other ways to make sure you are safe for driving, operating equipment, or doing other activities that demand high levels of cognitive function.

The journey of a thousand miles begins with a single step.

Chinese proverb

CHAPTER 4

Checklists and Routines

Form good habits. They are just as hard to break as bad ones.

In Chapter 3, you read how important it is to manage energy and prevent fatigue. To that end, nothing helps me with this process more than following routines and using checklists. In addition to saving needed cognitive energy for other tasks, routines and checklists cut down on mistakes and their associated frustration. I have used routines and checklists less formally since my childhood. I honed the skill with my training in medicine and aviation. Before my traumatic brain injury (TBI), using them made my life flow more smoothly. Now, I believe they make my comfortable and productive life possible. Where they were once a convenience, they are now a necessity.

The aviation industry has successfully used checklists and routines for many years. To reduce errors resulting in aviation incidents and accidents, this method of using checklists and routines has been moved to an even higher level of importance over the last decade or so, along with efforts to improve the communication skills of teams working together in aviation. The medical profession has also begun to embrace the use of checklists and routines, to prevent the tragic mistakes that have made front-page news. For example, the use of checklists and routines prior to surgery, including reviewing the planned surgery with the patient and the surgical team in the operating room prior to putting the patient to sleep, is lessening the frequency of such medical errors.

You can standardize some activities of your daily life, so that little cognitive energy is involved in doing them. *Routines* are generally unwritten ways of doing things consistently the same way. You may want to write things down initially, make a checklist, and follow it until the steps become automatic. *Checklists* are designed to be written, with each item on the list (usually in order of when it should be performed), either verbally "checked" off or actually checked off in writing.

Whether a routine or checklist will serve you better depends on the level of cognitive impairment you have. If you have poor memory, attention, and sequencing skills, written checklists, with every step spelled out, is likely best. If you have less impairment, simply outlining the activities to be done may be adequate. Do as much as you need to do to help you function efficiently and accurately.

For many activities, you can start with a checklist; then, if the activity is simple and straightforward, as you remember the items of the checklist, it can become a routine for you—an unwritten checklist.

Making It Through Your Day

♦ **Be consistent** in your daily schedule.

— Set a standard time and procedure for routine tasks.

— Your body and mind actually function better with consistent times for sleep, waking, and meals. We have a natural internal rhythm, and having a very erratic schedule puts more stress on us.

Getting Up

♦ **Wake up.** Try to get up in the morning about the same time every day. Set an alarm to help you awaken on time.

♦ **Shower.** Have a shower routine (whether done in morning or evening.) You need this if, like me, you forget whether you washed your hair or not. I'm sure I've frequently washed my hair twice, and I'm sure at times missed doing it completely before starting my routine. Now, I get in the shower, get wet, wash my hair immediately, and then wash my body.

♦ **Breakfast.** Fix breakfast the same way, at the same time each day. The menu is boring, but it gets this chore done without a lot of drain on precious cognitive energy! Use different cereals or types of bread for toast, but stay consistent, so that you do not have to spend cognitive energy making decisions about what to eat. I also set things out the night before if I have to leave the house early in the morning.

♦ **Pack a lunch.** The same thing applies to packing a lunch for the workday. The same lunch daily means fewer things to keep track of as far as buying groceries goes—and again, less thought. This is boring, but effective. This can also be done the night before.

Leaving Home

♦ **Make a schedule.** Figure out what you need to do on a daily basis before leaving the house, and make up a checklist or routine to deal with the process most efficiently and accurately.

Coming Home

♦ **Stash your stuff.** As you enter the house, put things away where they belong. This is very important, especially because you're often tired after a long day, and the inclination is to just set things down and go take a nap. The problem is, later you may not remember where you set things, or you may not remember to do something that needed to be done on arriving home. You may not have the energy or time later to put things away, so you slowly build a house full of clutter. Some specific things that need immediate attention upon arriving home include:

— Keys

— Glasses

— Mail

— Check voice messages

— Write down any to-do things that came up while away from home

End of the Day

♦ **Prepare for tomorrow.** Have a routine or checklist to prepare for the next day. Some possible items include:

— Set out your clothes the night before, so you have an easier morning.

— Pack your lunch.

— Set out your breakfast things.

— Pack your briefcase/backpack with what you need for tomorrow's activities.

— Make up a to-do list for any things you need to get done the next day.

♦ All of these simple routines, done the night before, make for a smoother morning and more energy left for your day's activities.

Trip Planning

♦ Make an agenda. Make up checklists or have routines for managing some of the following more complex activities associated with travel:

— Making reservations for lodging, airline, rental car, shuttles

— Trip/vacation packing

— Camping:

— Packing camping gear, clothing, food

— If using a camper, or even a tent, set up and tear down checklists are helpful

Managing Finances

Paying Bills

♦ **Pay bills automatically.** The best bill-paying routine for minimizing cognitive energy demands is to set up as many bills as possible to be paid automatically. This can be done with most utilities through their customer service departments. An added advantage is that you do not have to spend money on stamps.

♦ **Let your bank pay the bills.** When the service is not available from the service provider, you can often set up automatic payments through your bank. You will still get a statement in time to confirm that the payment amount is correct, but it will be paid on time without you having to deal with it. For any bills that you are unable to set up direct payments for, several options exist.

♦ **Use bill-paying software.** If you use a computer-based financial package, put the payment in and have a reminder sent to you at a designated time.

♦ **Use Stickies.** A free, downloadable software program called Stickies allows you to have "sticky notes" placed on the home page of your computer instead of stuck all over the computer screen and your work area. When you use other programs, the notes remain in the background. I can keep checklists for my financial activities on my computer home page and check off monthly bills, deposits, and accounts needing balancing as they are completed.

♦ **Pay bills as they arrive.** Write out the check, put it in an envelope, and attach a note to the envelope reminding you when the payment is due. This should then be put in a conspicuous area, where you will notice it regularly and get it sent off on time.

♦ **Make annual payments.** Pay annually or semi-annually things such as insurance (car, home, and health) and property taxes. Sometimes doing this earns a discount, and it keeps you from having to keep track of things during the year.

♦ **Use escrow accounts.** Set up your homeowner's insurance and property taxes to be paid out of an escrow account, included in your monthly mortgage payments.

Depositing Checks

♦ **Use automatic deposit.** Arrange to have checks automatically deposited into your banking account if possible. There are several advantages:

— You do not risk having the check stolen from your mailbox.

— You do not risk misplacing the check in your home.

— The money is usually available faster than if you received the check through the mail and deposited it.

Balancing Your Checkbook

♦ **Use checkbook software.** For me, the easiest method of keeping my checkbook balanced has been to use a financial software program, such as Quicken.

♦ **Get someone else to do it.** If you have a trusted friend or family member, ask them assist you or (even better!) do this task for you.

♦ **Get the bank to do it.** Some banks offer help finding problems, but many charge for this service.

A person with a clear purpose will make progress on even the toughest road. A person with no purpose will make no progress on even the smoothest road.

Thomas Carlyle

CHAPTER 5

Attention

Thinking is easy, acting is difficult, and putting one's thoughts into action is the most difficult thing in the world.

Goethe

The ability to sustain attention is critical to cognitive function. We have to pay attention to initially gather information to put into our short-term memory. Having memory problems makes it harder to pay attention because you don't remember to stay focused or don't remember what you were thinking, saying, or doing. In addition to simply being able to maintain attention—whether for short or sustained periods—the brain also has other attention functions:

Focused attention. The ability to pay attention to something you hear, see, or feel. It is actually like perception, being aware of stimuli around you.

Sustained attention. The ability to maintain attention for an extended time with continued or repeated stimuli, such as pushing a button whenever you hear a noise or see a light, and continuing to do so for an extended time.

Selective attention. The ability to maintain attention despite distractions, such as pushing a button when you hear a particular noise or see a particular color of light, while ignoring different noises or colors intermingled with those you are to respond to.

Alternating attention. The ability to switch between totally different activities, such as having a dinner conversation in a restaurant, getting interrupted by a question from the waiter, and returning to your conversation right where you left off.

Divided attention. This is the highest level of attention. It involves being able to simultaneously do multiple tasks. An example would be driving while talking on the cell phone.

Eliminate or Minimize Distractions

♦ **Keep it quiet.** Have important meetings and conversations in quiet places with minimal people movement around you.

♦ **Use background music**, preferable to talk radio, to drown out intermittent noises.

♦ **Use ear plugs.** Ear plugs or ear protectors can be bought in the hardware section of many stores. They are used for those working around loud noises to protect their hearing, but you can use them to block out any distracting noises.

Use a headset. Good-quality headsets or even better, noise-canceling headsets, with or without music can be helpful. Also, when you are wearing them other people tend to interrupt less.

Use a filter. Some people with brain injuries have difficulty filtering out background noises that went unnoticed prior to their injury. Ear filters are provided by audiologists. A mold is made of your ear canal and a filter is designed to fit your needs, based on hearing testing. The testing determines what level of sound filtering gives you the best discrimination (the ability to hear spoken words in the midst of background noises). By filtering out some of these background noises, you hear "better" despite actually hearing "less."

Eliminate clutter in your workplace. Clutter is very distracting to the mind.

Set up your workspace to minimize distractions. These distractions include windows, the fridge, and busy walkways in the home or office. Face your desk to the wall instead of to a window or hallway.

Practice redirecting your focus to get back on task if you find your mind wandering. This skill can be improved with practice. Talking to yourself, saying "keep focused" may help, especially when driving in busy traffic.

Turn on your answering machine, and don't answer calls when trying to get work done.

Put a "Do Not Disturb" sign on your door, close it and talk to family and co-workers about what that means.

♦ **Go invisible.** If you're working on the Internet, and you're signed up for instant messaging or voice over internet services, designate that you are unavailable or pick the "invisible" option.

♦ **Avoid overstimulating environments.** If you struggle with filtering issues—an inability to filter out extraneous auditory or visual stimuli—avoid going to very stimulating environments. Consider watching a DVD or video at home with friends rather than going to a movie theater. Or, consider having dinner in a small, quiet restaurant rather than at a large, noisy one. You may want to go for a hike in the woods rather than to a noisy bar with friends.

♦ **Take care of basic needs.** We all have a hard time paying attention when we are tired, hungry, or need to go to the bathroom—even without a brain injury.

♦ **Set a clear goal or objective** in your mind for what you are doing, preferably written down on a schedule or paper in plain view, as a memory jogger. This will help you return to your task after being distracted.

♦ **Write it down.** If you are told to do something, or think of something you want to do or remember, do it now or write it down. With any distraction, you may not be able to remember the information or come back to it later.

♦ **Highlight.** When reading material for retention, use a highlighter to help keep your attention, as well as letting you know where you left off if distracted.

♦ **Use notes.** When speaking from notes, follow your notes with your finger, so that if interrupted with a question you can find where you left off.

♦ **Try medication.** Some people with brain injuries benefit from the use of medications similar those used by people with attention deficit disorder. These medications help the brain stay on track. You should discuss this option with your physician to see if it fits your situation.

Improve Attention with Communications

♦ **Use cues.** If you have trouble with focused or sustained attention, consider having family or co-workers use key words to help you maintain attention, such as using your name; ask you to listen or look as appropriate; and maintain eye contact with you or touch you to keep you focused.

♦ **Get it in writing.** Ask for important information to be given in both oral and written forms.

♦ **Say it again.** Family and co-workers can ask you to repeat back what you've been told.

♦ **Answer questions.** When presenting, ask the attendees to write down their questions, so that they can be dealt with at the end, because interruptions make it difficult to keep on track.

♦ **Focus on the other person.** When in a distracting environment, maintain eye contact, sit close, and if necessary even ask the person you're talking with to slow down so that you can keep your attention focused.

Light Distractions

- ◆ **Wear cool shades.** Wear dark glasses to minimize bright light exposure.

- ◆ **Wear a visor.** Visors help when distractions are caused by bright lights or flickering fluorescent lights.

Everyone who got where he is had to begin where he was.

Richard L. Evans

CHAPTER 6

Memory

All improvement in memory consists of one's habitual method of recording facts.

Dr. William James,
Father of American Psychology

Memory impairment is a nearly universal issue for people who have had traumatic brain injuries (TBIs). Remembering new information is usually the most significant deficit for people with TBI. Most people with brain injuries have more problems with immediate (few seconds) and short-term (few minutes to hours) but not long-term (few years) memory functions. Many medical conditions affect memory as well as factors such as aging, fatigue, stress, depression, loss and grief, inactivity, not paying attention, interference/distraction, lack of organization, medications, vision and hearing difficulties, alcohol use, and poor nutrition.

Memory is not simply one function. To remember something, several processes must happen. First, we have to notice something. This involves concentration, or paying attention. Second, we have to store this information in the brain. We store information better if it is related to something we already know, or it has stimulated an emotional response. Last, we must be able to recall the information at a particular moment when needed. The more frequently we use a particular piece of information, the easier it is to retrieve. With memory deficits, any or all of these steps may be impaired.

I have trouble with attention/concentration, because I'm very distracted by things in my surroundings, even my own thoughts. As far as storing information, I like to compare my memory storage ability to Swiss cheese. Some things stick and are remembered, some things fall through the holes. There seems to be no relationship to how important something is and how likely I am to remember it. I'll remember the smallest detail and forget something of great importance. As far as the retrieval function, I like to say that my brain often likes to take the "scenic route" when trying to find a particular piece of information I need. Eventually, my brain will usually find it, but not generally within the timeframe I prefer.

Many of us who have had brain injuries have no difficulty with our long-term memory—remembering information stored prior to our accident. This is information we made an effort to remember, either consciously or unconsciously, because it was meaningful, important, or made an emotional impression. *Procedural memory* is also included in long-term memory. This is the memory of routines or skills you preformed so often that they became almost automatic. Many people don't even need to think to use the skills involved in the physical process of driving, riding a bike, skiing, and for me, flying my airplane.

After having done these activities hundreds of times, we have "muscle memory"—we just do the actions needed without conscious thought.

Sometimes, the information in long-term memory cannot be retrieved at the moment we want to access it, but it *is* there and it *will* come to us in time.

For most people with TBI, the real problem is in laying down new memory, creating new long-term memories from recent events and activities. Researchers found that many of the "mental exercise" treatments used to train the brain only help in the short term for memory problems. Memory retraining is labor intensive and not very effective over time. Trying harder to have a better memory is not a strategy that works, either.

For longer-term memory improvement, compensation strategies work best. Many of these strategies make memory "external." When I was still a practicing physician, I would tell my patients who wondered how doctors were able to remember the vast information available in medicine that I didn't need to personally remember every medical fact. I only had to know where to go to find it. That is the key to unlocking your memory.

With the help and support of therapists and families in learning to use memory-improving strategies and tools, as well as regular reminders to continue to use these tools, your memory will work even better. It takes time and energy to learn to use tools and strategies to compensate for memory impairment. The needed effort to use these strategies and tools becomes minimal once they are mastered and regularly used; they become almost second nature.

According to research, three main factors must be consider in improving memory function:

♦ We remember something better when all of our senses are involved—how it feels, sounds, looks, tastes, and smells.

♦ We remember things better that are of interest to us, not when boring or not applicable to us.

♦ New information is easier to remember if it can be "hooked" onto something we already know.

Improving Your Memory Function

Memory, like muscle coordination and strength, is a "use it or lose it" function. Brains that are worked regularly are better able to process and remember new information. It has been shown that increased television watching is related to declining memory as well as poorer overall health. To exercise your brain, you need to do new and different things. Simple things like changing your routines can help. Consider trying to write or brush your teeth with your left hand occasionally if you are right-handed. You can also do exercises that force you to use your faculties in new and different ways, like getting dressed or navigating around your house in the dark, or with your eyes closed. (Make sure you are safe when you do this, but challenge your senses.) Changing your route while driving or walking, even if you need to use a back-up map or GPS for safety, helps exercise your brain, as you need to remember new landmarks, process new information, and function out of your usual "groove." Realize that this brain exercise will use up energy, so pace yourself and don't plan this for a day already filled with other cognitive demands.

Reading and writing stimulate your brain. Learn new things; mastering new activities you've not done before stimulates neuron activity. This can include introducing brain teasers into your life such as card games; crossword puzzles; crafts; art activities; learning to dance, play an instrument, or speak a new language; or cooking new and different foods.

- ♦ **Take care of yourself.** A healthy lifestyle is important for cognitive function. You will remember things better after a good night's rest than when you are sleep deprived. If you are distracted and stressed by things in your life, you will not receive the information in the first place, let alone be able to put it into storage. Some medications impair memory— sleeping pills and pain medications, among others—so limit or eliminate anything in this category if possible. Maintain good habits, including avoiding smoking. Smoking leads to vascular disease, which can affect memory as well as increase the risk of brain injury from strokes.

- ♦ **Relax.** Avoid trying to force yourself to remember the information you want. Trying hard to remember something makes you frustrated, further worsening your capacity to recall something. Move on to something else, and often the information will appear to you.

- ♦ **Exercise your memory.** Your memory will function better if used regularly. Reading helps the processes involved with memory, including focusing or paying attention, organizing information, and remembering and retrieving information.

Iron rusts from disuse; water loses its purity from stagnation and in cold weather becomes frozen; even so does inaction sap the vigors of the mind.
Leonardo da Vinci

Memory Enhancement Techniques

♦ **Take a mental snapshot.** Visualize what you want to re-member. See a name written, even read the letters one at a time as you "see" them. Exaggerate the image with bright col-ors, added sounds or smells, or remember it as bigger than life. The more vivid the "picture" associated with what you want to remember, the more likely you are to remember it.

♦ **Pay attention.** It takes about 8 seconds' focus to move something into our memory center. Therefore, don't try to multitask when needing to remember new information. You might try mentally cataloguing something you are doing to help your memory. Say to yourself "I am setting my glasses here, and when I need them again I will return here to get them." It moves that action from being unconscious to con-scious. Actively observe and tell yourself what landmarks are around where you park your car, as well as how things look as you enter the store. My brain injury support group friend who does this also—as a back-up—engraves his name on his tools in case he still forgets where he puts them. It also makes sense to put your name on or in your things, so that they can be returned to you if you leave them somewhere.

♦ **Repeat.** Rehearse information, such as a name, to help it to be transferred into long-term memory. We all remember using flash cards in the past for remembering things. Now, I make cards of information I want to learn, such as new Spanish words. I carry them with me and, when I have spare time, review them repeatedly.

♦ **Chunk information.** Instead of trying to remember the 10 digits of a phone number such as 1372945869 as just 10 numbers, chunk them into 137-294-5869 and you are more likely to remember them. This also works for short lists.

♦ **Use cues,** such as the visual image of your phone sitting in your driveway when you need to make a call when you return home. When you see your driveway, you'll be reminded of the call. Many people remember speeches by associating each part to objects in a room of their house, or landmarks along a running or driving route. As you rehearse, visualize the objects or landmarks with each part of the speech to help you remember it.

♦ **Use word associations.** We all remember "spring forward, fall back" for how to reset our clocks twice a year. I take a word I regularly have a hard time recalling and attach it to some other word that has something to do with it. For some reason, the word "draft," meaning following in the slipstream of a vehicle, always gives me difficulty. I have associated it with a horse—"draft horse"—and usually can come up with it when needed now.

♦ **Use rhymes.** Many of us use "thirty days has September..." You can make a rhyme out of a name you're trying to remember, or even an extended rhyme out of a short list of groceries you need to pick up at the store.

♦ **Use acronyms.** ROY G. BIV is used to help schoolchildren remember the seven colors of the rainbow; Red, Orange, Yellow, Green, Blue, Indigo, and Violet. In flying we use C GUMPS for preparing to land; Carburetor heat, Gas (fuel pump on), Undercarriage (landing gear down), Mixture (gas/air ratio adjusted properly), Prop (propeller adjusted if applicable), and Seatbelts (all in plane have belts on). We have many other acronyms we use in flying to help us keep track of procedures when things get busy.

♦ **Use environmental cues.** Change something (which wrist your watch is on) or add something (a string on your finger) to remember something you need to do at a later time.

♦ **Keep things visible.** Putting objects in a conspicuous place helps remind you to take or use them. When I visit a friend and remove my jacket, I often hang it on the door knob, so that I don't leave without it. I will put something on the floor by the door to remember to take it or on the driver's seat of my car to remember an errand when I drive off. I'll also set my keys on things to take when I leave, or put a note on my jacket.

Compensating for Impaired Memory Function

♦ **Write it down.** My mantra is "Do it, write it or forget it." This includes plans, reminders, even thoughts.

♦ **Take note of your notes.** Put notes in a consistent place. It doesn't help to write notes to yourself that you cannot find later when they are needed.

♦ **Use a personal digital assistant (PDA).** Because we are not always home, having a scheduler, calendar notebook, or PDA to carry with us at all times is very helpful. There are many brands, or you can develop you own, but having one is essential:

— Write all appointments here.

— Carry a list of important contacts with their phone numbers and addresses as needed.

— Carry your scheduler/planner/PDA with you at all times when away from your home, and keep it in a convenient, readily accessible location in your home.

♦ **Write detailed notes.** Many complain of finding notes with just a phone number or a name that means nothing. If you don't write enough, so that someone who has no idea what you're writing about would understand it, you're at risk of not remembering what it means at a later time. Include in the note *when, where,* and *what* to make it more complete and useful.

♦ **Write down key words** and special information and mentally rehearse information. This is something I use with flying. Intermittently, I need to talk on the radio to other pilots in the air, to airport personnel, or to air traffic controllers. I have all the words I need in my brain, but sometimes I can't find them when I need them. To improve my chances of accurate communication, I write down the key words I need to say and, at times, even rehearse what I plan to say so that I get it right. I will use this same technique before making a phone call and before an important conversation.

♦ **Post it!** Use brightly colored sticky notes to move key information into your long-term memory. These are helpful, for instance, to prevent the problem of buying something new, putting it away in your house, and later not being able to find it.

— Put the information, in enough detail to later understand what it means, on a brightly colored sticky note.

— Put the sticky note in a very conspicuous place, such as on your refrigerator or bathroom mirror.

— When you see and re-read the sticky note every day (even better, read it out loud a couple of times), you will eventually move that information to your long-term memory.

— To be safe, consider then putting the note in your home journal, so that you can find it later if needed.

◆ **Keep a home journal.** A home journal gives you a place to write down things that are important and need to be remembered pertaining to your home. You might want to keep track of the names and numbers of repairmen, when they are coming if needed, what things you've done to your home or yard, and what things you might need to do. You can also keep track of the outcome of calls, including who you talked to and when. Consider using a three-ring binder, so that you can make separate tabs for different information. This journal stays in your home, to be available when needed.

◆ **Use dry-erase boards, blackboards, or bulletin boards.** Have these strategically placed around your house for writing reminders and keeping track of information. The benefit of dry-erase boards is that you can use differently colored pens for different levels of importance. An easy system is to use red, yellow, and green, like a stoplight: red for the most important information, green for the least. Put your reminder board:

— On the refrigerator. Handy for grocery lists and schedules of people in the house.

— Near the back door. To list things to be sure to remem-

ber when leaving the house and to write last-minute reminders.

— Near the computer. To jot down information quickly,
write yourself reminders, note information to include
in e-mails, and make to-do lists for computer use.

— Near the telephone. As a calendar with plenty of space
for writing notes and dates. Be sure to transfer information from here to your daily planner/scheduler if needed away from home or to coordinate your schedule.

♦ **Ask for help.** Reminder calls from offices where you have
scheduled appointments can be very useful. The call will
prompt you to keep the appointment on the right day and
arrive on time.

How to Prevent Losing Small
Often-used Items

Keys, glasses, and other smaller objects are easy to lose, and
frustrating hours can be spent looking for them when needed.
To prevent this, consistent strategies need to be used.

♦ **Have a consistent place for your keys** and *always* put them
there:

— On a peg near your front/back door

— In a small basket hanging on the doorknob

— Clipped to your purse/backpack

— On a lanyard around your neck or hang it over the door
when you are home

♦ **Use your keys to help remember other things** you need to take when leaving the house. Set things on a shelf near your back door, with the keys on top, so that you don't forget them when leaving. Or, attach your keys to your backpack or briefcase when away from home, so that you don't leave it behind.

♦ **Have a consistent place for your glasses:**

— In a small basket

— In an eyeglass holder

— On a chain/cord around your neck

Finding Things You Have Put Away

Do you often put things away in the "right place" or in a "safe place" in your home, office, workshop, camper, or any other place you spend your time, only to have no idea where they are later, when needed? This is especially important if you rearrange things, move, get a new camper (my issue), or are staying for extended periods away from your home. Make use of the brightly colored sticky note tip previously mentioned and make sure you are consistent in putting things away where they belong.

♦ **Label it.** Put labels on drawers, doors, cabinets, and boxes listing the enclosed items.

♦ **Sort it.** Where you have large shelves or drawers available, consider sorting things used for similar activities into smaller baskets or clear bins.

♦ **Have a miscellaneous basket.** If needed, have one basket, shelf, or area for putting things that don't have an official place until you can decide where that place should be.

Medications

♦ **Use a pill organizer.** Pill organizers work well for remembering to take medications. If needed, you can either use an alarm or you can buy pill organizers with alarms built in to remind you to take medications at different times of the day.

♦ **Keep your organizer filled.** Fill the organizers (consider using several weeks' worth) and check the number of pills remaining. If you are getting low, put the needed order date into your scheduler.

♦ **Keep meds visible.** Put the pill organizer in a place where it will be readily visible as a reminder. Next to your bathroom sink works for morning or evening dosing, on the kitchen counter or table near where you eat for dosing during the day.

♦ **Take your pills with you.** Have a small medication carrier to take with you if you are going to be away from home at the time medication is needed, and consider using an alarm for a reminder.

Memory Tools

Calendar/Schedulers

♦ **Use a calendar.** Calendars are helpful for keeping track of appointments. A small and portable one can be handy to have when away from home to remember appointments and add new ones. Cross off activities/days after completed.

♦ **Use a calendar/organizer.** These are more elaborate book-type calendars with sections to keep track of personal information, contacts, medications/medical information, and to-do lists as well as other important information.

♦ **Use your PDA.** A PDA is an electronic organizer containing a calendar, contact storage section (often with notes), to-do list section, a calculator function, and more.

— In studies with patients who had had brain injuries, PDAs were found to be more effective in remembering activities/appointments than written forms of organizers due to their alarm functions. This was true even if family or caregivers had to input the information.

— PDAs can synchronize information with a computer. This allows information to be inputted into the computer, rather than the PDA itself. It also allows sharing schedules with others easily. Calendars can also be printed for posting if desired.

— With a PDA it is easy to put in repetitive appointments or tasks, entering them once and having them repeat at their needed interval.

— A disadvantage may be the difficulty of easily seeing a week's or month's activities at a time to better plan activities and avoid overwhelming your energy stores.

— If you are a new PDA user, start with one function at a time and develop competency before taking on another function, to avoid being discouraged by the technology.

♦ **Use a paging system.** NeuroPage systems are available that link to your computer and page you, reminding you of appointments, time to take medications, and other activities.

Copier/Scanner

♦ **Copy it.** Copy and file all medical, insurance, and legal papers.

♦ **Scan it.** With a scanner, you have the potential to scan documents and save them in your computer rather than in a paper form. This technique is for confident computer users, and it requires adequate computer back-up to avoid loss of critical information with a computer glitch.

♦ **Copy your recipes.** Copy recipes, so that you can check off ingredients and steps as you do them.

♦ **Copy sewing/craft patterns.** When I knit, I copy the pattern, so that I can write on the copy to keep track of where I am on the project.

Digital Camera

You can use the one in your cell phone (if available) or use a separate one to help you remember things.

♦ **Take a picture of your car.** Take a picture of your car, where it is parked, row numbers, and landmarks.

♦ **Take a picture of something you need to buy.** This allows you to select the right type, size, and color at the store.

♦ **Take a picture of something you see** to remember it later.

♦ **Take a picture of new people** you meet to put in your file system with their name to help remember them.

♦ **Take step-by-step pictures.** With severe memory impairment, pictures can be taken of steps to a procedure, such as making coffee, to allow a person to complete the procedure independently.

Digital Voice Recorder

♦ Use a digital voice recorder to record information when note taking is not possible or efficient:

— Key chain recorders that will hold 20 to 60 seconds of input are good for short messages, car location, and other brief notes.

— Digital recorders are available with extended memories for meetings, conferences, class notes, noting things while driving, and more complex notes.

Labeling Machine

♦ **Label everything.** Labeling doors, shelves, bins, boxes, and drawers helps you find things, but also helps you to return items to their proper place after use.

— Label closet doors with the categories of items enclosed.

— Label shelves with items stored on them.

— Label bins/boxes/drawers with enclosed items.

Telephone and Answering Machine

♦ **Use your answering machine as a memo recorder.** Call when away from home and leave yourself a message. Many machines also have a *Memo* button that you can press to record a message while at home, either for yourself or for someone else in the household.

♦ **Keep writing materials near your phone** to take notes as needed.

♦ **Program emergency and frequently called numbers** into your phone.

♦ **Prominently display needed contact numbers** near the phone.

♦ **Write out directions** to get to your house, and post them near the phone to provide to callers if needed.

Keys

♦ **Set up a key holder.** Place a key holder or key safe with a PIN number outside your house or car, in case keys are lost. Or, leave a key with a trusted neighbor.

♦ **Color code keys** with tags/key colors to make it easier to find the right one.

♦ **Keep keys handy.** Have a consistent location for all keys.

Learning to Use New Technology

♦ **Break it down.** For any technology or complicated process you need to learn, break the process down into steps. You will do better if you break new techniques down into manageable bits, and master one before moving on to the next.

♦ **Read the instructions.** To manage the amount of material given in instruction manuals, here is a suggested process:

— Skim the manual to see what general information it contains.

— Use a highlighter to highlight areas of particular interest/need.

— Figure out what functions you need, and look at those particular areas first.

— Attach labeled tabs to the manual on important pages to quickly and easily find them later.

— If needed, write up a list of needed procedures on a card you can carry with you.

Technology makes everybody's lives easier, but it makes people with disabilites' lives possible.

CHAPTER 7

Time Management

Though I am always in haste, I am never in a hurry; because I never undertake any more work than I can go through with perfect calmness of spirit.

John Wesley

Many who have had brain injuries report that their concept of time is off, maybe because everything takes longer to do. In the past, you gauged the passing of time by what you had accomplished. You can have difficulty staying on time because you can be distracted by so many things and get off track. Everything seems to take longer to do, so if you don't plan in extra time, you're always running late.

Many people with traumatic brain injury (TBI) also get more fatigued than they used to, especially if they have done any mental activity or had any emotional issues to deal with. You need more sleep at night now, and you need to rest and take more breaks during the day if you have been very cognitive. This significantly decreases the productive time available to you in a day. You also may notice that you now have lower stress and frustration tolerances than in the past. All these things must be taken into consideration as you plan your days.

In response to the complaint that "I don't have enough time for something," the truth is that we all have the same amount of time in a day and that we make choices every day on how to "spend" our time, just as we choose how to spend our money. We cannot truthfully say we do not have time for something, but we must admit that we do not choose or plan to spend the time we have on that activity.

We always have enough time if we use it right.
Goethe

Managing Your Schedule

♦ **Use one tool at a time.** Try to use only one calendar, scheduler or personal digital assistant (PDA) to keep track of your schedule and information. When you use more than one tool, you risk missing things, double-booking yourself, and increasing your work load. Carry your calendar with you at all times.

♦ **Use a simple calendar.** Use a calendar with no more than one block per hour and plenty of space for writing information.

♦ **Set a date.** Be sure to move things from the daily to the weekly or monthly calendar, whichever you use for advance planning.

♦ **Check your schedule** on the weekend, before the start of a new week to plan out your week and avoid surprises concerning appointments or time commitments you have made.

♦ **Check your schedule again** the night before for early morning commitments, in the morning to plan your day, and regularly throughout the day to keep things from slipping through the cracks.

Personal Digital Assistant Tips

♦ **Schedule reminders.** When you enter an appointment, schedule a reminder enough in advance to prepare for the appointment, usually by several days.

♦ **Change the reminders.** When the reminder comes, change the scheduled reminder to enough time to make it to the meeting, allowing time to get ready and to travel.

Written Calendar Tips

♦ **Use a highlighter.** On a paper calendar, use different colors of highlighters to signify different types of activities. This allows you to see at a glance what types of activities you have within a given day, week, or month. Activity types to differentiate include medical or other appointments, work, fun activities, classes or seminars, and things you don't want to forget, like birthdays, anniversaries, and the like.

♦ **Prioritize your activities.** Look at the activities that take up your time. Are they activities that are worth this valuable commodity? Maybe some, such as television time, can be decreased to allow more time for other activities, such as exercise.

Besides the noble art of getting things done, there is
a noble art of leaving things undone. The wisdom
in life consists in the elimination of nonessentials.

Lin Yutang

Managing Your Day

- **Stick to the routine.** Set a standard time and procedure for routine tasks.

- **Do it over...and over.** Fix breakfast the same way every day at the same time. The menu is boring, but it gets this task done without a lot of drain on your day's cognitive energy. The same applies for packing a lunch for the workday. The same menu and routine also lets you to know how long to plan for the activity.

- **Do it the night before.** Set out what you need for the day the night before. This saves time in the morning and helps you to not forget needed things.

- **Stick to your schedule.** Commit to making it work, and avoid distractions.

- **Turn off the phone.** Avoid wasting time with unnecessary phone calls from telemarketers and your cousin Harry.

- **Limit e-mail.** Avoid logging onto your e-mail account unless it is in your schedule to do so.

- **Don't think about what is next** or tomorrow.

I never think of the future, it comes soon enough.

Albert Einstein

Getting Things Done

To-Do Lists

A to-do list can help organize your time and budget your energy in a number of ways. A list can

— Give you a readily visible idea of what you want to accomplish

— Give you a place to write odds and ends of things you want to accomplish

— Reinforce the mantra of "Do it, Write it, or Forget it"

— Free up your memory for things that you do not need to be working hard to remember

— Help you prioritize your goals for the day, week, month, and even year

♦ **Jot it down.** Keep a place handy, maybe in your calendar, to jot down things you think of that need doing throughout the day. At this point, you only need to note the activity, not its priority, complexity, or importance.

♦ **Make up a schedule.** From this master to-do list, you can make up your weekly schedule, including all things you hope to accomplish within that week.

♦ **Categorize your to-do list.** Consider separating your weekly schedule's to-do list into categories, such as yard, house, work, and financial, and monthly and weekly repetitive activities, such as taking out the trash.

♦ **Make a template list.** Keep monthly and weekly repetitive items on a template list, to make list making more efficient each time.

◆ **Make a daily list.** From your weekly schedule, you can plan your daily to-do list.

◆ **Break tasks down.** Instead of putting "clean office" on the list, put "clean the in-box" or "clean off desk surface." This makes the task more manageable in time and effort, giving you a better chance to accomplish it. It also helps with sequencing, as you can put down the steps in order and cross them off as completed.

◆ **Schedule tasks.** Schedule a task to be done at a particular time, with both a start and stop time. This helps keep you on track during a day, and also prevents you from spending hours on a task and burning out.

◆ **Use a computer.** If you are good with the computer (or if you have someone who can help you), make up a weekly schedule template, with set times for things such as going to bed, getting up, meals, exercise, rest, housework, and fun/entertainment.

◆ **Block in the time.** Fill in blocks of time to work on your to-do list items.

◆ **Plan for energy use.** Plan more cognitively challenging activities for the morning and least cognitive activities for later in the day.

◆ **Fill in the blanks.** Pick a time on the weekend to fill in any upcoming obligations for the week in your template, and then you can fill in any other specific things you want to schedule. Then print the weekly schedule.

◆ **Pencil it in.** Each day, set aside a time to pencil in your to-do time blocks with items from your weekly/monthly to-do list.

◆ **Set an alarm.** Consider an hourly chime on your watch or an alarm to let you know when it is time to start something and—just as important—to let you know when it is time to finish. Working for hours on something is often nonproductive, because you become tired and your frustration level rises as you make more mistakes.

♦ **Limit major activities,** like repairs to make on your house. Consider limiting this list to three items, and only add a new item when a previously listed item is either completed or removed from the list.

♦ **Prioritize.** Assign a priority to all items on your to-do list, either by color coding the text on the computer before printing or using a highlighter. The stoplight colors—red for critical, yellow for important, green for less important—are easy to remember.

Timers and Alarms

♦ **Use your watch.** Consider using a watch with hourly chimes, which can remind you to check your schedule and see what you are supposed to be doing for the next hour. The hourly reminder also gives you a better idea of the passage of time during a day, even when you are not following a schedule.

♦ **Get a multiple-alarm watch.** Watches are available with up to three alarms that can be set during a day for reminding you of necessary activities. Without an alarm, or at least an hourly chime, you may find yourself working on a project until the wee hours of the morning. This makes it difficult to perform well the next day, and for days afterwards.

♦ **Use your kitchen timer.** Kitchen timers come in different, very convenient forms. You can get an electronic one that is very loud, easy to set, and magnetic, so that it can be attached to your refrigerator where you can find it when needed. Some kitchen timers also have a lanyard (most of these are also magnetic), so that you can keep the timer on your fridge, then take it with you if you leave the area and need an alarm to remind you of something.

♦ **Use a vibrating timer.** Some timers are pager-sized devices in which you can set multiple alarms in a day, as well as a repetitive alarm to go off at regular intervals, such as every hour. You can set the alarm to be audible, or you can set it to vibrate so you don't disturb those around you when it goes off.

♦ **Alarm your PDA.** When you enter planned activities in your PDA, set the alarm function. Consider a self-imposed rule to never shut off the alarm on your PDA without either doing the activity immediately or resetting the alarm. Otherwise, without fail, you will get distracted and forget that you have an appointment in an hour or two.

♦ **Be realistic.** You must be realistic about how many things you can actually accomplish in a day. Better to succeed with fewer planned activities than to fail with too many. As you are more successful with managing your time, you can add more cognitive activities to your day.

♦ **Start low and go slow.** Unless you wake up in the morning feeling as rested as you did the morning before, you overdid it yesterday and are not ready to add more to your day. Many of us are in a hurry to return to our preinjury level of activities, but we need to start low and go slowly, gradually building up the amount of activities we undertake in a day. Success will breed more success as well as motivation. Failure will breed frustration and anxiety, both of which worsen cognitive function.

The main thing is to keep the main thing the main thing.

Stephen Covey

CHAPTER 8

Organization

The definition of insanity: doing the same thing over and over again and expecting different results.

Albert Einstein

Prior to my traumatic brain injury (TBI), I had a reputation of being a very organized person. I organized my time, my surroundings, and my finances with great skill. I had learned the basics from my mother when growing up, and through my schooling, medical training, management training, and training as a pilot had fine tuned these skills and considered myself a master organizer. Not everyone is organized, but those who are tend to work in more complex jobs requiring a high degree of multitasking. Multitasking requires good skills in dividing and alternating attention, managing time, communicating effectively, having good memory skills, and preparing yourself well for planned activities. These skills were all impaired to one degree or another after my brain injury. As a result, I found myself floundering, trying to make it through the simplest tasks, let alone trying to be productive in my life.

My previous style of accomplishing things—working hard and long—didn't seem to be very effective helping me to manage the chaos of my life. Trying harder to "be organized" also doesn't work very well; it's similar to trying harder to hear when you are deaf, or to see when you are blind. However, this doesn't mean you can't become organized, just as you can learn to communicate when you are deaf and navigate your surroundings when you are blind using strategies and tools you can learn.

To be organized, you need to draw on all of the strategies and tools you have already learned thus far. You can organize time (your day, week, and month), spaces (your bathroom, kitchen, and wardrobe), and things (your papers, calendar, finances, and mail). It is an ongoing process, and the skill of organizing yourself can be fine tuned as you take on and master new strategies for dealing with attention, memory, time management, communication, and routines and checklists.

Entire books have been written on organizing your life, and there are people whose occupation it is to help others get organized. Many strategies and tools are available, some that work for everyone, some more tailored to individual needs. This book can't begin to cover all of the possible strategies and tools, but I'll try to provide information on many that you can use. It is a good place to start; as with any other strategy and tool, organization strategies and tools only work if used. It is not easy to change the habits of many years, but it can be done.

How well we recover from our brain injuries depends on who we are—our attitudes, work ethic, ability to ask for and use help, and our ability to accept and even thrive on change. Our recovery is an ongoing process. We will, at times, have setbacks, need new strategies and tools for changes in our lives, and have available to us new technologies as they are developed.

> *The journey of a thousand miles begins with a single step.*
>
> Chinese proverb

Organize Your Time

Time management was covered in detail in Chapter 7. The tools we use to organize our time will help us to organize the rest of our lives, including our spaces and things. Some key points are repeated here, along with some new ones.

Use a Scheduler/Planner/PDA to Keep Track of Activities

♦ **Write it down.** Write every planned activity and all task lists in it to have them available at all times.

— Sit down weekly with your schedule and plan out your week.

— Sit down daily with your schedule and plan out your day.

♦ **Review your schedule.** Check your schedule regularly throughout the day, so that you don't forget things and you keep on task. If you have trouble remembering to do this, set an alarm as a reminder.

♦ **Carry your schedule with you.** It will do you no good sitting on your desk when you are at a meeting and need to schedule an appointment.

♦ **Use only one schedule.** Try to use only one schedule to avoid forgetting to transfer things between schedules. When you try to work with multiple calendars, invariably some appointment, meeting, or other obligation will slip through the cracks by getting written on one of your calendars but not on the one you are using at the moment.

♦ **Plan your trips.** When making trips away from the house, try to list all planned things to accomplish on the trip so none are missed. Consider the times businesses open and close when you plan your route. Even consider ordering stops for the most efficient travel route. This will make the best use of your time and also cut down on mileage costs.

Meetings

♦ **Write the dates of meeting and any deadlines in your scheduler.** If the deadlines are on dates different from the meetings, put them in your schedule also.

♦ **Keep information for meetings in folders.** If needed, note in your scheduler that you have a folder of material to remember to take to a particular meeting.

♦ **Remind yourself of responsibilities.** Write any actions you are responsible for and reminders for them in your scheduler.

To-Do Lists

♦ **Prioritize the list.** Use the stoplight colors, red, yellow, and green, or use letters or numbers to prioritize tasks.

◆ **Break big items down** into smaller items, and do one step at a time. A large project seems daunting to many who have had brain injuries. By breaking it down into smaller steps, it is not as unwieldy to handle, plus you can order the steps in sequence to increase efficiency.

◆ **Keep it short.** Long lists, like big projects, can be daunting.

◆ **Use alarms to start/end tasks.** Spending too much time on the same project can lead to frustration and inefficiency as mental and physical fatigue set in.

◆ **Do one thing at a time.** Most people who have had brain injuries have a diminished ability to multitask. It is better to do one thing well, than two or more things poorly. This is especially true with more complex tasks, like cooking or dealing with finances. Try to find uninterrupted time and space to do these things.

◆ **Allow more time for activities.** The reality is that we *do* get distracted, have trouble with initiation, and get easily fatigued. Set realistic goals. Stretch your abilities, but not to the point where you are failing regularly and getting frustrated and anxious. As you find you are succeeding, you can raise your expectations. Someone getting a new artificial leg doesn't expect to run a marathon right away, although that might be a realistic long-term expectation.

◆ **Reward yourself** for progress made, and make sure to include fun in your schedule. Keeping yourself healthy emotionally, which includes having fun, allows you to continue to maintain a good work ethic. You need to have something to look forward to, not endless hours of difficult work.

People rarely succeed unless they have fun in what they are doing.

Dale Carnegie

Organize Your Spaces and Things

♦ **Organize yourself.** Important key strategies will help you stay organized in your day-to-day activities. Being organized helps compensate for any memory deficits, saves time looking for things, lessens your daily cognitive energy demands, and allows you to accomplish more.

♦ **A place for everything, and everything in its place.** Put your things in the same place *every* time. This includes your keys, glasses, wallet or purse, scheduler, planner, or PDA, and other items you need to use on a frequent basis. This will save you hours of time and much frustration spent looking for things you need on a regular basis. Assign a place for nearly everything, and commit to putting things there. Also encourage those around you, including family, friends, and co-workers, to honor those assigned spaces for your things.

♦ **Unclutter your space.** If you are a "collector" or a "clutterer," seriously consider attempting to "de-stuff" your house. Clutter causes problems with attention and saps your energy. With fewer possessions, you have fewer things to keep track of and care for.

♦ **Pick up and put away.** Plan time in your schedule every day for picking up and putting away things, and do it. It is easiest to put things away when you use them, but the reality is that things pile up. If you are consistent in working to "declutter" every day, you will have an easier time than trying to deal with a house that has become filled with piles on every horizontal surface.

Bathroom

♦ **Use it or lose it.** "De-stuff" by getting rid of any bath/beauty/hygiene products you haven't used in six months and of expired over-the-counter or prescription medications.

♦ **Put what you use daily in a conveniently accessible place;** consider putting the supplies in a basket to keep them all together.

♦ **Store less frequently used items** in the cabinets/cupboards in clear or labeled containers, so that you can find them easily.

♦ **Assign a space for each family member's items.**

♦ **Use shower caddies** for holding items needed in the shower, and install hooks on the back of the door or over the shower door for towels.

Kitchen

♦ **Throw it out.** "De-stuff" by getting rid of any food products that are outdated or appear spoiled. General guidelines for storing food:

— Canned foods (2–5 years)

— Cereal (6 months)

— Condiments (1 year)

— Dried herbs (6 months)

— Flours (3–6 months)

— Grains and legumes (1 year)

— Pasta (1 year)

— Spices (6–12 months)

♦ **Put what you use daily in a conveniently accessible place;** consider putting the supplies in a basket to keep them all together.

♦ **Store less frequently used items** in the cabinets/cupboards in clear or labeled containers so you can find them easily.

♦ **Store things to be visible and accessible,** as well as making the best use of space:

— Use divided drawers, small storage shelves, and clear storage containers for storing similar items.

— Chose containers that are square and stackable to take up less space.

— Use pull-out wire bins in deeper cabinet shelves, and bins that allow cans to be stored on their sides and roll forward as each preceding one is used.

♦ **Keep non-kitchen "stuff" out of the kitchen.** The kitchen is often the room people come into first, and everything gets dropped there to remain for eternity.

Wardrobe

♦ **Hang it up.** To start de-stuffing your wardrobe, turn all of your clothes hangers around, then turn them back when you wear the item. If the item is never worn in a season, consider discarding it.

♦ **Throw it away.** Discard any worn, stained, or unmatched clothing, like single socks. Consider if you really *will* mend a torn item, shorten or lengthen something, or fix a zipper. If it is not likely, get rid of it. Discard shoes with worn heels or insoles, as these can increase your risk of a fall. Consider discarding running or walking shoes when you've put 400 miles on them, even though they may look good yet. You are again increasing your risk of injuries due to unseen support deterioration.

♦ **Keep items you actually wear,** that fit, and that can match with other clothing and accessories easily. Then, when shopping, consider carefully whether you really need that new blouse, pair of pants, or shoes. Buying less clothing not only keeps your wardrobe more manageable, but saves you money.

♦ **Separate clothing** into work/dress and casual, so that you can quickly find what you need for either activity.

♦ **Use color-coded hangers.** You can put work and casual clothing on different colored hangers to make picking out clothes fast and easy.

♦ **Sort clothes by color.** Sort your clothes by color, to make matching outfits more efficient.

♦ **Store out-of-season clothing.** Try to move out of season clothing to a storage area. I have a cedar closet in my basement, where off-season clothing can be stored for easy access when switching seasons. This also makes the clothing accessible for any trips to climates that are different from mine.

♦ **Move nonclothing items**—suitcases, accessories, and the like to another space.

Home De-cluttering

♦ **First things first.** Pick the space that bothers you the most to work on first.

♦ **Schedule a time,** preferably when you are fresh, to undertake the task.

♦ **Ask for help.** Consider asking a family member/friend for help.

♦ **Begin sorting.** Get a couple of boxes/bins and a trash container. Label the bins to designate what you want to keep and what you want to get rid of, either by selling or donating. Sort things in the space you are de-cluttering into "keep" and "get rid of" (possibly separated into donate, sell, and trash).

— Dispose of the trash.

— Mark and set aside stuff to be donated to take to a local thrift store on your next trip out of the house, or call and schedule the items to be picked up at your home.

— Put away the stuff to keep in the place you choose.

♦ **Label it.** If rearranging cupboards, cabinets, and drawers, consider labeling them with what types of items they contain so you can find things easier in the future. This is especially true when you bring new items into your house or put old things away in new places. The space that made so much sense will not seem so obvious tomorrow or next week when looking for the item. If storing things in containers, attach labels with the contents listed, so that you don't have to open them to know what is inside.

Office Workspace

♦ **Limit horizontal surfaces.** The more you have, the more places available to make "piles."

♦ **Label** all of the drawers, cubbyholes, and crannies, so that you can find things as well as know where to put them after use.

♦ **Work ergonomically.** On a healthy note, make sure your desk and chair are set up so that you are working ergonomically. When sitting up straight in your chair:

— Your arms should hang loosely with your elbows bent at 90 degrees.

— Your forearms and thighs should be parallel to the floor.

— Your back and calves should be perpendicular to the floor.

— Your feet should be flat on the floor.

— You should be looking straight ahead at your monitor.

— Your eyes should be focused about one-third of the way down from the top of the screen.

— Your wrists should be flat or slightly cocked up on the keyboard and mouse, definitely not bent down.

Finances

♦ **Use automated bill paying.** Set up automated bill paying with companies whenever possible. If available, use your bank's automated bill paying service.

♦ **Use pay-date reminders.** Put reminders in your scheduling system for bills that can't be paid automatically. You can also use a desktop Stickies program for this, which places a virtual "sticky note" on your computer's desktop that lists your credit card due dates. Each month, change the font color from red (unpaid bill) to green (paid bill) for easy reminders.

♦ **Use a financial software package.** These programs are big timesavers and increase accuracy. You can set up reminders for monthly bills, pick how many days in advance to be reminded, download statement information from banks and credit card companies, as well as organize information for tax preparation.

♦ **Pick two days a month to work on paying bills,** whichever works best for you. Put this in your scheduler as a recurring activity.

♦ **File your bills.** Put all bills to be paid in a specific place and, after they are paid, file them in folders by month or by category. Category examples are auto, insurance, utilities, and mortgage. Use whichever works best for you.

♦ **Save tax receipts.** Make a folder marked "income tax" and place any bills and receipts that you need to keep track of for your tax preparation in that folder.

♦ **Toss unneeded paperwork.** Shortly after the first of the year, go through your financial folders and dispose of anything from the previous year that you no longer need. Anything needed for tax preparation should be moved to your tax folder.

♦ **Limit credit cards.** If you use only one, then you have only one credit card bill to keep track of each month.

Ask for credit card fee waivers. Credit card companies are sympathetic to an occasional misstep, so don't be afraid to call them and ask for waiver of fees. This won't be granted if it is a common occurrence though.

Paperwork

Handle it once. Deal with papers once: either file them or dispose of them.

Use In and Out boxes. If you just can't do this, have "In" and "Out" boxes. The "In" box is for mail, bills, and papers that must be dealt with. The "Out" box is for items that are completed and need to be filed.

Use labeled file folders. Make file folders labeled for all your common household bill-paying categories, but also for common things you need to keep, such as car and house papers, insurance policies, TBI material, professional licenses or certificates, and the like.

Color code your files. Consider color coding your files, with different colors for finances, work, school, medical, or other major categories you need. It is easier to find a misplaced file this way.

File alphabetically. Arrange files in each file drawer alphabetically, to make them easier to find.

Index your files. A file index can be kept on the file cabinet or in front of each drawer.

Use subcategory folders. When a subcategory is needed, and depending on how many papers it will hold, you can either use a manila folder in the hanging file or put another hanging file behind the main one with a different colored label on it.

♦ **Computerize your documents.** Set up your computer document files as folders, using the same system to make electronic file storage consistent and easy to manage.

♦ **Clean out your files.** Yearly, usually in January, go through your files and clean out any outdated or no longer useful information. Talk to your accountant or tax preparer and attorney about how long you should keep financial and legal papers.

♦ **Get a fireproof safe or safe deposit box.** Keep important financial and legal records in a fireproof safe or a safety deposit box. Make sure someone in your family or a close friend knows where these papers are and how to access them.

Mail

♦ **Sort it.** Whoever sorts the mail should divide it into stacks or bins for each person, with whoever is responsible collecting all of the household-related mail. Sort incoming mail into four main categories:

— Things that need to be dealt with, such as bills, receipts, and letters to answer by mail or phone

— Things to file, such as insurance policies or receipts

— Magazines, catalogs, or letters that you want to read or letters

— Junk mail to shred or toss

♦ **Junk mail.** A joint decision can be made about junk mail, whether to just toss or shred it, or pass it along to the addressee.

♦ **Handle everything once.** The goal is to handle everything only once (or the least number of times possible). This cuts down on your workload both in handling incoming mail, finding important papers, and dealing with needed outgoing mail.

Tools for Organizing Your Life

Time

♦ **Use schedulers, planners, or a PDA** to keep track of your schedule.

♦ **Set alarms.** Set alarms, either on your clock, watch, or PDA, to remind you of when to start and stop activities.

♦ **Use a family calendar.** In the family setting, consider one posted calendar for family schedules so everyone knows who is or needs to be where and when. Color coding for each person helps you see things at a glance.

Spaces and Things

♦ **Use a backpack or briefcase for each different type of major activity,** such as work, exercise, rehab, or medical appointments if they are occurring often. Pack your bag in advance, with the items you will need. Attach clips or carabineers to it for attaching keys, to keep them from being misplaced and your bag from being forgotten.

♦ **Use file cabinets.** In your office or workspace, file cabinets are always useful.

♦ Use different colored files for each drawer or main category such as work, medical, finances, and the like.

♦ **Minimize desk surfaces.** Consider putting your computer in a hutch or armoire rather than on a table or large desk. This way, you minimize the horizontal surface for cluttering and have bins, drawers, and spaces to store the important things you need within easy reach.

♦ **Shred, recycle, or toss.** Have a paper shredder, recycle bin, and garbage can in your office to dispose of no longer needed papers and unneeded mail.

Cooking

Cooking can be a challenge to anyone with memory impairment and attention issues, or to anyone who is just trying to do too many things at once. Who hasn't forgotten to shut off the stove, burned something in the oven while answering a phone call, or had a pot on the stove boil over?

♦ **Set a timer.** Make it a habit to never turn on a burner or the oven without setting a timer for when things should be checked. You can use regular timers as well as those attached to cords to wear around your neck. With the timer on a cord, you can carry the timer with you if you leave the room, so getting distracted won't lead to ruined food or a fire.

Recipes

Your ability to follow a recipe may have significantly changed since your brain injury. You may have trouble with "details." You may have trouble remembering if you added an ingredient or how many cups or tablespoons you've already put into the pot or bowl. You may not follow the sequence in the correct order or seem to miss important steps in the recipe. Sometimes it isn't critical, but it's not easy to grease a pan *after* you put the batter in it.

♦ **Break it down.** Break down a recipe into steps.

♦ **Assemble ingredients.** Get all ingredients out and onto your work surface before starting.

♦ **Measure everything first.** Measure each ingredient into a separate small dish, bowl, or measuring cup. This way, if you're not sure you put in all that is called for, you can re-measure. If you accidentally put in two tablespoons instead of two teaspoons, you can dump it back into the container and remeasure.

♦ **Stow it.** After you've measured out an ingredient, put the container away.

♦ **Check it off.** Check off each ingredient as you add it to your bowl or pan, and check off each step as you do it. (Make a copy of the recipe first, so that you can write on it.)

♦ **Make time.** Because of the added time needed to assure you follow the recipe correctly, make sure to leave yourself enough time to finish the recipe.

♦ **Do ahead.** If you are going to have limited time in the morning or after work to make something, measure out all of the dry ingredients ahead of time, put them in a covered bowl on the counter, and set any tools or cookware needed to make the recipe out on the counter. Make sure refrigerated ingredients are measured and readily available in the morning.

♦ **Plan a weekly menu.** Sit down on the weekend after making up your weekly schedule and plan what you will be fixing for meals during the week. On busy days, plan to eat leftovers, make simple meals, or have someone else cook. On less busy days, plan to cook a bigger meal. By knowing what you plan to make, you can figure out any groceries you might need for the week also.

♦ **Cook in advance.** When you have time and energy available, consider making meals up in advance and freezing them to have meals available when you don't have the time and energy to cook.

Shopping

The entire process of shopping is fraught with issues for those who have had brain injuries. These issues include remembering what you want to get and where you parked your car; dealing with the visual, auditory, and smell sensory overstimulation that some have problems with; and managing the fatigue that comes from coping with these issues. Some strategies to make shopping easier are included here.

♦ **Pick the time of day to shop that suits you best.** Consider going early, when stores are less crowded and you are more alert.

♦ **Make lists.**

— List what you want to buy. Make the list as complete as possible, with item, amount, even brand if that is important.

— Make up or purchase standard shopping lists that contain commonly needed items. You can do an inventory before leaving home and see if you need any of the items, and how much.

— Consider shopping for a few items each time and shopping more often if overstimulation or fatigue are significant issues for you.

♦ **Get someone else to do it.** If you have serious issues with shopping, consider getting someone else to shop for you. Some stores offer this service to their customers. You also can order things online in some stores and pick the order up at the store to limit time spent in the store.

Grocery Shopping

♦ **Make a master list.** To save time on this repetitive task, consider creating a master list. This can be done on your computer, and then edited for each planned shopping trip. You can even arrange the list by how your usually visited grocery store orders its isles. Put some staple items on the list permanently, and leave spaces to write in other more intermittently needed supplies.

♦ **List it as you finish it.** Have a notepad or dry-erase board on your refrigerator to write down anything you need to replenish. Make it a house rule that the person using the last or next to last of an item must write it on the refrigerator list.

Housecleaning

This job can be overwhelming, but you have options: hire someone to do the housekeeping for you, or do it yourself, in steps and stages. If you live with others, divide up the duties.

♦ **Break it down.** If doing housework yourself, break down the duties into manageable steps to do daily, weekly, monthly, or yearly as needed to cover all needed areas.

Daily Cleaning

♦ **Avoid clutter.** Pick it up, put it away!

♦ **Clean up while cooking.**

♦ **Stack the dishwasher.** After eating, wash or put dishes in the dishwasher and empty when done.

♦ **Use spray cleaners and disinfectants** for shower or tub, spray each time after use.

♦ **Use automatic toilet bowl cleaner** to minimize the cleaning needed.

Weekly Cleaning

♦ **Carry supplies with you.** Keep your cleaning supplies in a bucket/carrier.

♦ **Do things in order.**

   — Dust first. Disposable dusters are nice to use—no clean-up afterward.

   — Sweep and then dust mop any hard surface areas.

   — Vacuum house.

   — Mop any floors needing it.

Seasonal Cleaning
"Spring Cleaning,"
"Pre-Holiday Cleaning"

We all need to do seasonal cleaning to spruce up the house for the holidays, or to freshen things up for spring.

♦ **Make a list.**

   — Wash windows, clean screens, clean window coverings.

   — Wash indoor trim and doors.

   — Wipe down walls.

   — Wipe down inside of kitchen and bathroom cabinets.

   — Move out and clean under and behind large appliances.

   — Clean refrigerator and freezer, oven, microwave, and stovetop.

   — Clean lint out of dryer vent.

   — Have carpets and furniture cleaned and stain-protected.

   — Straighten storage areas.

Home Maintenance

This is another big job that can easily overwhelm you. You have the same options as with housecleaning: hire someone to do it, or do it in steps. And, if you live with others, you can divide up the duties.

Spring

♦ **Make a list.**

— Replace furnace and air conditioning filters.

— Have heating and air-conditioning systems serviced.

— Replace smoke and carbon monoxide detector batteries.

— Check for winter water or ice damage to attic, walls, foundation, roof, basement.

— Inspect outside of house including trim and doors/door frames for paint or wood cracking.

— Check seals on doors, windows.

— Clean and install window screens.

— Make sure gutters and downspouts are cleaned out.

— Inspect and repair caulk, seal around sinks, tubs, showers.

♦ **Consider a service contract** with a heating and air conditioning company. They'll contact you when routine service is due and take care of seasonal furnace and air conditioner duties.

Summer

♦ **Replace furnace and air conditioning filters.**

♦ **Perform water heater maintenance.**

— Drain any sediment and water.

— Refill.

— Check that temperature is set at safe level. A safe recommended temperature for hot water is 110° F.

— Check pressure valve and vent for proper functioning.

♦ **Inspect for and repair or replace any loose roofing shingles.**

♦ **Inspect for and repair any driveway, sidewalk, steps, deck, or porch damage.**

Fall

♦ **Make a list.**

— Replace furnace and air conditioning filters.

— Replace smoke and carbon monoxide detector batteries.

— Check seals on doors, windows.

— Remove and store window screens.

— Remove window-mounted air conditioners.

— Cover and disconnect evaporative coolers.

— Remove hoses from outdoors, and drain underground sprinkler systems if in areas that freeze.

— Consider shrinkable plastic seals on windows for winter if more insulation is needed.

— Inspect and repair caulk, seal around sinks, tubs, showers.

— Have heating and air-conditioning systems serviced.

— Inspect any unvented gas heaters for proper ventilation.

Winter

♦ **Make a list.**

— Replace furnace and air conditioning filters.

— Make sure gutters and downspouts are cleaned out.

— Make sure sump pump is functioning properly.

— Inspect attic, garage, outbuildings for rodents or other pests.

♦ If you live in an area of the country with winter snow, place shovels, snow removal equipment, and ice removal products in an easily accessible location.

Laundry

Like cooking, laundry can be a challenge even for those without cognitive dysfunction. A load gets put in the washer, something distracts you, and days later you find a dried out mass of clothes. You forget a load in the dryer, and everything is full of wrinkles. Here are some tips to make laundry easier.

♦ **Set a timer.** Set a timer when you put things in the washer. Use one on a cord around your neck if you will be wandering away and unable to hear an alarm from the laundry area.

♦ **Leave the lights on.** If the laundry area is in your flow of traffic moving around your house, leave the light on to serve as a reminder whenever you are doing washing or drying.

♦ **Limit the number of loads** to how much time you have to do laundry.

♦ **Finish what you started.** Try to finish what you start, all the way to folding and putting the clothes away, if possible, so that you don't leave more clutter in your house.

If we fail to plan, we plan to fail.

CHAPTER 9

Communication

Remember that our worth and value are not wrapped up in what we can do. We are not human doings, but human beings.

I t is reported that one of the main reasons relationships end, both personal and business, is from a lack of good communication. People without brain injuries or cognitive dysfunction have plenty of communication problems, so when you add the challenges of dealing with deficits from a brain injury, communication issues become an added barrier to establishing and maintaining close relationships.

Speech and Language Basics

Researchers have encouraging findings in the area of language and communication. They have discovered that language and communication problems can continue to improve for a long time after the initial injury. This is true for spelling, arithmetic, and speaking. People can also continue to improve in their ability to understand things they have read or heard.

The cognitive or thinking aspect of communication can be affected when the *receptive function* (listening/reading) and/or *expressive function* (talking/writing) is impaired. Many of us with brain injuries have subtle hesitations in our speech as we search for a word or the meaning we wish to convey, or we try to figure out where we were heading in a conversation. We also sometimes miss the meaning of what someone was telling us, either from not understanding what they meant, not paying attention to what they said, or losing part of long or complex conversations due to short-term memory deficits.

◆ **Work with a speech therapist.** Speech therapists can help people with brain injuries see their areas of strengths and challenges. We can learn *compensations*—new ways of doing old things—that help us make up for some of our language problems. Finally, the practice and feedback that speech therapists give in therapy sessions can lead to better conversation skills in social situations, too.

◆ **Use e-mail.** Some people with brain injuries report that they prefer communicating via e-mail rather than in telephone conversations. With written communication, you have more time to organize your thoughts and plan what you want to say and how you want to say it. When you talk with someone on the telephone, without fail, something you had intended to tell them was forgotten, you forget to ask something you wanted to know, or you make plans for a time already scheduled with another activity. When using e-mail, you can also plan your communication times for when you are rested and ready, not when the phone happens to ring.

♦ **Join a brain injury support group.** Among people with similar cognitive challenges, you will feel less conspicuous with having less than perfect communication skills. You will see immediately that you fit in, and that others in the group "get it" concerning the challenges you are dealing with. Members of support groups also share information about the people who have helped them, tools they have found helpful, and issues they continue to struggle with.

♦ **Check out the 'Net.** Programs are available on the Internet or to be used on home computers to work on speech and language. To find them:

— Consult with your speech therapist or special education teachers at local schools.

— Search the Internet for Web sites and products, for example, Bungalow Software products, available at *www. bungalowsoftware.com.*

Processing Verbal and Visual Information

I find that, since my brain injury, I seem to listen and communicate mostly on one level only. I have trouble getting the multiple meanings of jokes, sarcasms, and some figurative expressions. I take everything literally, as my brain doesn't seem able to process what is being said while I'm hearing it—it just sends it through verbatim. Some people with brain injuries do not always filter what they say, as they seem to not be able to think about what they want to say or how they want to say it as they are speaking. I also find that if I don't catch the first few words in a sentence, the entire sentence ends up sounding like gibberish to me. It is like my hearing of the information gets off track and can't get back on track. This is especially true in group settings with background noise or when I am tired.

With short-term memory issues, many of us have significant problems when given instructions that consist of more than one step. When the second or third steps are given, the previous information is lost. What seem like simple instructions to those giving them are frustrating for us—we usually end up looking for something to write with or we try to deal with the matter without using the instructions.

I can also see changes in how I process visual information. I may see a road sign, recognize all of the words, but the concept escapes me. I may substitute words in what I read and have difficulty figuring out what is going on. I often find that after I read a sentence or paragraph, it didn't register, and I can't remember what it was I just read.

Some report that it takes a lot of concentration to stay focused in conversations and while reading for retention. They need to stay hypervigilant, similar to when they hear a noise in the night and really focus to listen for it again. They need to maintain that level of vigilance while talking, reading, and especially while driving, in order to receive and process the incoming information.

♦ **Slow down.** When talking, slow down and try to give yourself time to think before speaking. Little pauses while you think before replying are usually not noticed by others, or they think you are giving an idea some thought before responding. This is so much more comfortable than the typical conversation, in which someone starts talking before the other person is even finished. It also helps to maintain eye contact with the person you are talking to. Much of what we get out of conversations comes from nonverbal communication. Facial expressions and body language add information to what is actually being said. This is one of the reasons that I like to talk in person rather than on the telephone, where I don't have access to this added information.

◆ **Rehearse.** Say what you want to communicate to yourself and see if it sounds right. If you are planning an important conversation, practice the important points in advance, even if it means writing out notes.

◆ **Repeat.** Repeat back what you hear, paraphrasing it, to see if you really understood what was said. Ask clarifying questions, to be sure you understand exactly what the other person is trying to say. Don't be afraid to ask the person you are talking with to slow down and stick to one topic or idea at a time to help you better participate.

◆ **Avoid distractions.** Have important conversations in quiet, nondistracting places and at times when you are least tired. Definitely avoid important conversation in the car while you are driving. Not only will you not be able to participate fully, you will be increasing your risk of an accident.

◆ **Get it in writing.** Ask for instructions and needed information in writing.

◆ **Read aloud.** Read things out loud to help you pay attention and better retain the information.

Tools

◆ **Carry a note pad** with you so that you can write down information or instructions.

♦ **Carry a digital recorder** for complex instructions, memory items, or for recording important information.

♦ **Use a highlighter.** Some find using highlighters when reading helps them to retain the important points, plus highlighting allows them to find key points faster in the future, if the information is needed again.

Word Finding

Not being able to find a word when you need it is a common and very annoying problem. It is not strictly a memory issue, but more a filing and retrieval issue. You know the word or name you want, but it cannot be found in your brain "file." It is similar to having all the files in your file cabinet emptied on the floor. Every piece of information is there, but finding it can be a challenge. To one degree or another, word finding problems are thought to affect almost every person who has had a brain injury. People who have never had a brain injury have occasional word finding problems, but those with brain injury face this issue more frequently.

Many of us become very proficient with *circumlocution*, describing or "talking around" an object instead of naming it. For many of us who have this problem, it affects self-esteem and self-confidence because we are not sure of ourselves when speaking. For some occupations, it can be a significant impairment.

Along with not finding a word, some who have had brain injuries have issues with word substitutions. You will mean to say one word but instead insert a word that often has nothing in common with what you wanted to say. At times, the words are similar, for example "I can't keep my thoughts on train" instead of "on track." It can be seen in writing too. Some substitutions sound the same, some are totally different words. Sometimes you realize you've substituted a wrong word, sometimes you're unaware of it. The interesting thing is that often these substitutions are not noticed by others, as they are getting the "gist" of the conversation instead of listening to every word. Sometimes it makes for a funny situation.

Work with a speech pathologist/therapist to learn techniques to decrease word finding problems. Some techniques used include:

♦ **Use circumlocution.** Describe the object you're trying to name instead of naming it.

♦ **Recite your A, B, Cs.** Go through the alphabet to see if a letter triggers finding the word.

♦ **Picture it.** Try to visualize the spelling or writing of the word.

♦ **Relax.** The harder to force yourself to come up with the word, the more frustrated you get and the worse you function.

♦ **Write it down.** In situations where using correct words is critical, such as communicating on the radio while flying, write down the key words so that they are in front of you if needed.

♦ **Use word association.** For words or names you continually "misfile" and can't find, try to come up with a word association, something that reminds you of the word or name.

♦ **Write a script.** Try "scripting" something important that you want to say. Either write it out or practice it beforehand, so that you get it right.

♦ **Play word games.** Doing crossword puzzles and playing

word finding games may help your brain become more efficient at filing and retrieving words.

Concentrating

For some of us with brain injury, the ability to concentrate or organize our thoughts is impaired. We may be easily distracted by things in our surroundings, so that we cannot concentrate on what is being said. We may forget something we heard or wanted to say and, in trying to think of what it was, not pay attention to what is being said. We often start to say something, only to forget what we were attempting to get at or "where we were going." We also tend to interrupt others, trying to avoid forgetting what we want to say in the flow of the conversation. All these factors affect our ability to stay involved in conversations. These tips can help make concentration easier.

♦ **Pick appropriate times and places** for important conversations:

— Avoid noisy, busy locations.

— Seat yourself where you will be able to limit traffic and noise around you.

— If you have them, wear your ear filters.

— Avoid times when you are tired.

— Limit the length of the meeting to a manageable duration, considering your available cognitive energy.

♦ **Ask for an agenda** in advance to prepare for the meeting.

♦ **Take brief notes** of things you want to remember or what you want to say.

♦ **Ask another person** present to take notes or record the important points being discussed.

Don't talk and do at the same time. If you have trouble concentrating and paying attention, then trying to do something while conversing, in person or on the telephone, sets you up for problems. Give the conversation you are involved with your undivided attention.

Don't talk and drive. Because of the attention and concentration required in a conversation, do not attempt to talk on your cell phone while driving. Driving is cognitive enough without diluting your attention with a conversation. Pull over if you need to make or answer a call.

Communication Tools

Cell Phone

Do not use a cell phone while driving. Even consider turning it off, so that an incoming call doesn't distract you at a critical moment.

Program frequently used numbers.

Use a voice-activated system for calling, if you have one.

Telephone

Use portable telephones, so that they can be conveniently located.

Use a headset. Consider using a headset to help with hearing conversations when distractions are present.

♦ **Program your ring tones.** If available, set up different rings for programmed numbers, so that you can quickly and easily have an idea of who is calling. That way, you can decide whether or not to answer and be prepared for the conversation.

Answering Machine

♦ **Screen calls** so that you can deal with a call when you are prepared, alert, and have the needed information readily available.

♦ **Ask for phone numbers and information** to be left slowly.

— Use the memo function, if available, to record memos for you or for family members.

— When you're away from home and need to leave a reminder for yourself or others in your home, call and leave a message on your answering machine.

Computer

♦ **Set your font preferences.** You can change the color, size, and appearance (font) of the print on your screen, as well as the color of the background, to make it easier for you to read. You can also choose settings in most e-mail programs to affect the size and color of the font and the color of the background in outgoing and incoming e-mails. For your regular computer activity, this control is in the *Display* folder, found in the *Control Panel*. The Control Panel may be an icon on your desktop, or it can be found by going to the *Start* screen. In your e-mail program, look for the word *Set-*

tings somewhere on the screen.

E-mail

Without care, dealing with e-mail can consume all of your waking hours. These tips will help:

♦ **Set up specific times** during the day to check e-mail. Avoid checking e-mail continuously during the day.

♦ **Set an alarm** if needed to limit this time.

♦ **Don't set up an incoming e-mail audible alarm** to tempt you to deal with e-mail at other than planned times.

♦ **Deal with an incoming e-mail once.** Read it, answer, file, or delete it and move on.

♦ **Set up files for important e-mail categories,** so that you can move e-mails out of the inbox to make the contents of the inbox more manageable. Regularly check and clean out your inbox and sent e-mails files to cut down on items you have to monitor.

♦ **Don't allow unimportant forwarded e-mails.** Request that family and friends not forward things on to you unless they are important.

♦ **Use the BCC option.** Ask those who send e-mails to you and others at the same time to use *blind carbon copy* (BCC) option, so that your e-mail address isn't sent on to others, and do the same yourself when sending e-mails to groups of people.

♦ **Don't open strange e-mails.** Do not open e-mails, especially e-mail attachments, from senders you do not recognize. These are at high-risk for viruses.

♦ **Ask people to reply to your e-mails** by including your original e-mail messages, so that you can remember exactly what you wrote.

Safety Issues

♦ **Carry personal identification** and emergency contact information on you at all times.

♦ **Carry medical information with you.** If you have any significant medical conditions, keeping detailed medical information, including names and doses of medications, next to your ID card is very helpful.

♦ **List your preferred emergency contact.** In your cell phone, planner/scheduler, or personal digital assistant (PDA), label your preferred emergency contact ICE, "In Case of Emergency."

♦ **When traveling, carry the name and contact information for where you are staying.**

You have brains in your head. You have feet in your shoes. You can steer yourself any direction you choose.

Dr. Seuss

CHAPTER 10

Transportation

*Planning is bringing the future into the present so
that you can do something about it NOW.*
                                        Alan Lakein, Author

Traveling locally or to distant places can be a challenge.
Travel requires the use of all of our cognitive skills: organization and sequencing, memory, energy and time
management, attention, communication, and reading and writing, and it also makes physical and emotional demands upon us.

Getting around, and doing it with the least amount of cognitive energy drain, requires attention to details. This is not an
area where "go with the flow" is a good idea. We can get lost,
overwhelmed, and even hurt if careful planning is not done rou-
tinely.

Driving is a very cognitive, energy-demanding activity. You
must pay attention to multiple things at once, process lots of
incoming information, think quickly, and make decisions rap-

idly. There are many distractions both in and out of the vehicle. Issues will arise that you are unprepared for, but if you plan as much as possible, you can minimize potential problems.

Getting Around in Your Town

♦ **Prepare in advance.** Make sure that you have all the needed information and supplies for your planned trip, even if it is only to the local grocery store.

♦ **Know where you are going.** Make sure you are familiar with the route, especially if you don't use one of the many Internet mapping programs available to look up directions. These mapping services can help you get to any location where you are not very familiar.

♦ **Plan your stops.** If multiple stops are planned, plan the best order to make drive time and energy use most efficient.

♦ **Avoid busy times and routes.** Consider the best time to go and which route to travel to avoid heavy traffic and busy intersections.

♦ **Minimize distractions.** If others are in the car, set rules for conversation to avoid distractions at inopportune times. Consider whether the radio is distracting. Music may not be, talk radio may be.

♦ **Check your vehicle before leaving.**

— Make sure you have plenty of gas for your planned trip.

— Walk around the car to make sure all of the tires are in good condition.

— If night driving is planned, check that the lights all work.

— Completely clear windows of snow, ice, and frost.

— Make sure you have change for a parking meter if needed.

— Have a local map in your car, as well as a compass.

— Make sure you have up-to-date registration and insurance certificates in your vehicle.

Traveling Away from Your Home Area

♦ **Use public transportation.** Consider public transportation when available, especially when going into urban areas. Consider this for a concert or sporting event, or when traveling to the airport.

♦ **Get someone else to drive,** even if you are taking your car. This is especially useful if you are going to an activity that has a high cognitive energy demand.

♦ **Car pool.** For a regularly scheduled activity, car pool. This not only cuts down on the cognitive energy you need for driving; it also cuts driving costs and allows for socialization.

Maps and Directions

♦ **Use an Internet-based mapping program to plan your route.** Consider using it even with familiar locations, if the driving will be cognitively demanding. These services give you a back-up if your brain gets overloaded, and they decrease the cognitive load of driving, leaving you with energy to do things at your destination.

♦ **Avoid major highways.** Some mapping programs have an "avoid highways" option. For many people with a traumatic brain injury (TBI), information processing is not as fast as pre-TBI. This option can be very helpful when keeping up with multi-lane traffic and road signs at highway speeds is not one of your better skills.

♦ **Buy a global positioning system (GPS).** If you do a lot of traveling or have to drive frequently to unfamiliar locations, a GPS makes it possible to travel more easily to unfamiliar places, especially in the dark when signs are difficult to read. It can give you the confidence that, even though you might get temporarily displaced, you are never lost. However, even with a GPS, consider still using a mapping program and always carry a map and compass.

♦ **Compare GPS information and maps.** Before a very involved trip, sit down beforehand and compare the GPS and mapping program routing to see where they might differ.

♦ **Check for construction.** Also check to see if any of the planned roads might have construction that may make them inconvenient to use.

Vehicle Contents

♦ **Bring food and water for the trail.** Whenever you plan to be away more than an hour, or even with shorter trips, carry water and snacks. If your pet travels with you, have water for him, too.

♦ **Carry a cell phone.** If you have one, carry a cell phone so that you can call a friend if needed for emergencies or even if you become too tired to feel safe driving. *Nothing that you do regularly is more cognitively demanding than driving.* Talking on a cell phone or doing other things while driving is very dangerous. Many studies have shown those of us who have had TBIs are more susceptible to driving accidents, for many reasons. Please do not add to the risks by trying to divide your attention.

♦ **Get a roadside emergency service plan.** You may be able to change your own tire, but would not want to have to do it in the dark or on a narrow shoulder near traffic. Emergency service plans also cover lock-outs and running out of gas, as well as providing a tow-truck service if your car breaks down.

Parking

♦ **Park in the same place.** When possible, park in a consistent location. If the parking lot is very large, or you will not be parking outside of the only entrance, park as closely in line with the *main entrance* as possible. For example, stand at the main entrance and look out into the parking lot. Imagine a wedge-shaped section—like a clock face, with the hands set at 11:00 and 1:00—with the point where you are standing. Park your car as close to 12:00 as you can. Then, when you come out of the building, you know that if you walk straight out from the main entrance, you will find your car. If you like to get as much walking in as possible, park far out in the lot. Your vehicle is usually found more easily, since it is not in a crowd of other vehicles.

♦ **Decorate your antenna.** If you have a small vehicle, or a common model and color, consider attaching something distinctive to the antenna, to attract your attention.

♦ **Take note of your parking place.** Sometimes, you don't want to use the main entrance, or a main entrance isn't obvious. Or, perhaps you will be parking in a garage with multiple levels. In these cases, note taking is essential to not losing your car:

— Write down your vehicle location information in your personal digital assistant (PDA), planner, or scheduler or on a note.

— Record it on a digital recorder.

— At the airport parking lot, put your parking slip in with your tickets and itinerary and place it in your carry-on travel bag.

Traveling For Extended Periods

Trip Planning

♦ **Use a travel agent.** Consider using a travel agency or tour company for any more involved travel.

♦ **Look at location and timing.** If, like many who have had brain injuries, you do not do well with overstimulation, try to plan trips to popular destinations during the "off season."

♦ **Think about the kind of trip you are planning.** If you are light sensitive, going to a sunny beach does not make a lot of sense. If crowds overwhelm you, a large cruise ship or gigantic amusement park may not be a good destination. Considerations should be given to climate, congestion, health care availability, available rest opportunities, and other personal factors.

Packing

♦ **Use a packing checklist.** If you travel often, develop a packing checklist for different types or lengths of travel. You can use your computer to print off the particular list you want, then check it off as you pack.

♦ **Organize in advance.** Organize what you want to take in advance, in a spare room or on the floor, using your trip checklist for reference. Make piles sorted by days for short trips, or by type of items—pants, shirts, socks, etc.—for longer trips.

♦ **ID your luggage.** In each piece of luggage, put a card carrying your name, cell and home phone number, and a contact address.

♦ **Color code your luggage.** Use colorful suitcase straps or other identifiers, so that you can easily pick out your luggage at the airport. These can be just regular straps, or lockable, using TSA-approved combination locks.

Special Considerations

♦ **Make a to-do list.** Start well in advance of the trip with a trip to-do list. You can use a dry-erase board; your planner, scheduler, or PDA; or your computer list to keep track of things you want to remember.

♦ **File it.** Set up a brightly colored hanging file in your desk file drawer or file cabinet for any papers, tickets, or travel information you may need for the trip. That way, everything has a place where you can find it later. Also put your passport in this file if it will be needed.

♦ **Copy your itinerary.** Make extra copies of your itinerary, with contact numbers for the travel agency, hotels, and other important information, both to carry along with you and to give to appropriate family and friends.

♦ **Carry needed medications with you.** For prescriptions medications, carry a copy of the original prescription, as well as the amount of medication you'll need to take during your trip. Carry medications in their original (pharmacy) bottles, clearly labeled.

♦ **Take it easy.** Plan a day or two without any obligations when you return home. This gives you a chance to unwind and also to get things put away from your trip.

The road to success is always under construction.

CHAPTER 11

Navigating the Medical Maze

I do not ask to walk smooth paths
Nor bear an easy load
I pray for strength and fortitude
To climb the rock-strewn road.
Give me such courage I can scale
The hardest peaks alone
And transform every stumbling block
Into a stepping-stone

Gail Broke Burket

I have spent time on both sides of the doctor–patient relationship. I had been told early in my training that if more doctors had to experience being patients, they would be better doctors.

Many of us who have had brain injuries do not volunteer information about how much difficulty we are having, even if we have the self-awareness to *know* how much difficulty we are having. We want to be as "normal" as possible, at the cost of propping ourselves up during the day and collapsing at night from the cognitive fatigue. We use up a lot of our daily allowance of cognitive energy trying to not appear "brain damaged," even when interacting with our medical professionals. Cognitive issues are invisible; you might not want to appear to be a complainer, but you have to tell your doctors and others about these issues in order to learn better how to cope with them.

Choosing a Medical Professional

♦ **Get a primary care physician.** These doctors provide the initial contact between the patient and the medical establishment. They accept responsibility for the continued care of the patient or family, and they perform a wide range of services. They serve as the quarterbacks of the medical system and may direct and coordinate activities they do not perform personally. They should be your advocate and guide through the complicated medical care system. For adults, a good primary care physician should be a family physician or internist (they practice adult medicine only.) For children, either a family physician or a pediatrician is best.

♦ **Find the right physician.** To find a physician, consider the following:

— Ask for references from friends and family members.

— Check with your state's Brain Injury Association to see if they have a referral network and if the doctor you're interested in is listed.

— Attend local brain injury support groups and ask for medical professional referrals.

♦ **Consider your criteria.** Look for a primary care physician who:

— Takes time to listen

— Takes time to talk

— Plans ahead to prevent problems

— Prescribes medicine carefully and reluctantly

— Reviews your total health program regularly

— Has your trust and confidence

— Is available, both for medical care and to deal with insurance and other forms and paperwork that will come up

The Medical Appointment

These tips will help with your medical appointments, but the information can be helpful with setting any type of appointment, medical or not.

Scheduling the Appointment

♦ **Consider timing issues:**

— Think about "better brain times" for appointments.

— For transportation, consider arranging a ride versus driving yourself.

♦ **Gather information in advance:**

— Office directions

— What do you need to bring?

— Are there any special dress requirements?

— Do you need to come early to first appointment?

— What are the payment options?

The Appointment

♦ **Make up an "Ask-The-Doctor Checklist"** and plan ahead for the visit:

— Make a list of symptoms or complaints.

— Make a list of any medications you are currently taking.

— If you have seen a doctor before for this problem, take the record with you if available.

♦ **Fill out the forms:**

— Plan to arrive early to complete forms, or ask for them in advance.

— Take all past medical-professional contact information with you.

♦ **Bring an advocate.** Ask someone who knows you well and whom you trust to accompany you to your appointment. Discuss your concerns and goals for the visit in advance so the advocate can help process the information given, ask questions, and help you remember what was discussed.

♦ **Tips for during the visit:**

— Avoid chit-chat; your time with the medical professional is valuable.

— Prioritize; state your main problem first.

— Describe your symptoms.

— Describe any past experiences with the same problem.

♦ **Get needed information for medications, tests, or treatments:**

— Ask for the name of the medication, test, or procedure.

— Find out why you need it.

— Ask about the risks.

— Ask about any alternatives.

— Ask what happens if you do nothing.

— Find out how to properly take the medication.

— Ask how to prepare for the test or procedure.

♦ **Ask questions.** Information to gather before the visit is over:

— Make sure you are given the diagnosis, or considered diagnoses (what's wrong).

— Ask if you need to return for another visit.

— Ask what you can do at home.

— Ask how to get the test results.

— Ask what signs to look for that are of concern and what might happen next, as far as your condition but also pertaining to planned tests, treatment, or follow-up.

— Ask when you need to report back about your condition.

— Ask if there is anything else you need to know.

The Patient's Responsibility

♦ **Educate yourself.** You must work to become educated about your own health and take care of yourself. Your doctor is a consultant to help you do this, not a caregiver to do it for you. Take advantage of the wealth of available medical information in books, newsletters, and on the Internet. You are responsible for your own health. No one is as concerned or passionate about your health as you are.

Perseverance is not a long race; it is many short races one after the other.

Walter Elliot

CHAPTER 12

Resources

If your ship doesn't come in, swim out to it.
Jonathan Winters

Education and information are some of the most effective tools available to help persons living with brain injury, as well as their family and supporters, deal with the resulting cognitive challenges. Those of us who know what might happen during the days, months, and years after our brain injury, how to understand it, and how to cope with it are likely to do better than those without this information. Therefore, accessing brain injury information early on in the process and when new challenges arise is very important.

I have listed many organizations and Web sites related to brain injury, disability, rehabilitation, and more. The information on these sites was correct at the time of writing; but, as we all know, Web sites, addresses, and phone numbers change. If

123

a site is not found at the listed address, try searching for it by name in a search engine. If unsuccessful, many other sites are available with excellent information.

Brain Injury Organizations and Agencies

Brain Injury Association, Inc.
Founded in 1980, the Brain Injury Association of America (BIAA) is a nonprofit organization dedicated to improving the quality of life of people living with brain injury, and their families, as well as promoting prevention of brain injury. The Web site provides information, education, advocacy, support, and prevention. The BIA consists of 42 state associations, 200 chapters, and over 800 support groups across the United States.

Many of the State BIA Chapters have extensive information on their Web sites and are worth checking out.

1608 Spring Hill Road, Suite 110
Vienna, VA 22182
Phone: 703-761-0750
Fax: 703-761-0755
Family hotline: 800-444-6443
Web site: www.biausa.org

Brain Injury Society
The Brain Injury Society is a federally exempt 501(c)(3) corporation committed to empowering persons living with conditions caused by a brain injury. The organization works with clients, families, and caregivers to identify strategies and techniques to maximize the new-found potentials for a stronger recovery. In this way, individuals recovering from brain injuries are better able

to lead active, productive, and meaningful lives while becoming as independent as possible in a rarely given second chance.

Brain Injury Society was created to offer a quick response service to all brain injured (whether acquired or traumatic, recovered and recovering) individuals. Acquired and traumatic brain injuries have overlapping symptoms yet are very distinct from each other. Acquired brain injury is an internal disorder caused by neuro-organic malfunctions. Traumatic brain injuries are externally caused, as in car accidents, sports injuries, and physical assaults.

Mailing & Billing Address Only:
1901 Avenue N - Suite 5E
Brooklyn, NY 11230
Telephone & Helpline: 718-645-4401
Web site: www.bisociety.org

Brain Trauma Foundation

The Brain Trauma Foundation was founded to improve the outcome of traumatic brain injury (TBI) patients by developing best-practice guidelines, conducting clinical research, and educating medical personnel.

523 East 72nd Street
8th Floor
New York, NY 10021
Tel: 212-772-0608
Fax: 212-772-0357
Web site: www.braintrauma.org

Dana Foundation/Dana Alliance for Brain Initiatives

A private, philanthropic foundation with principal interests in science, health, and education. The Dana Alliance, a nonprofit organization of more than 200 neuroscientists, was formed to help provide information about personal and public benefits of brain research.

745 Fifth Avenue, Suite 900
New York, NY 10151
Phone: 212-223-4040
E-mail: danainfo@dana.org
Web site: www.dana.org

Head Injury Hotline

Provides callers with information on living with brain injury, including consultations and referrals to health care, legal professionals, and support groups. Established by the Phoenix Project, a TBI information clearinghouse. Web site contains hotline information and an e-mail address.

212 Pioneer Building
Seattle, WA 98104-2221
Phone: 206-621-8558 (V)
E-mail: brain@headinjury.com
Web site: www.headinjury.com

The National Resource Center For Traumatic Brain Injury

Provides practical and relevant information, including videotapes. Develops educational materials including intervention and assessment tools. Web site contains lists of materials available, a question-and-answer column, and relevant links.

Department of Physical Medicine and Rehabilitation
Medical College of Virginia
Virginia Commonwealth University
P.O. Box 980542
Richmond, VA 23298-0542

Phone: 804-828-9055 (V)
Fax: 804-828-2378
E-mail: mbking@hsc.vcu.edu
Web site: www.nrc.pmr.vcu.edu

National Stroke Association
9707 East Easter Lane
Suite B
Centennial, CO 80112-3747
info@stroke.org
Tel: 303-649-9299 800-STROKES (787-6537)
Fax: 303-649-1328
Web site: www.stroke.org

International Brain Injury Associations

International Brain Injury Association: www.international-brain.org
The Brain Injury Association in U.K.: www.headway.org.uk
Brain Injury Association of Canada: www.biac-aclc.ca
Brain Injury Australia: www.bia.net.au
Brain Injury Association of New Zealand: www.brain-injury.org.nz
Irish National Association for Acquired Brain Injury: www.headwayireland.ie

Web Sites

Brain Injury Information Resources

American Academy of Neurology
Web site: www.aan.com

The Brain Injury Information Network
TBINET was started in 1995 by a small group of caregivers who had loved ones with various types of brain injuries. They developed a Web site devoted to helping people find information on ABI/TBI. Besides a significant resource directory, they have multiple support mailing lists covering brain injury, stroke, coma, Down's syndrome, etc.
Extensive resource list: www.tbinet.org/resources.htm
Web site: www.tbinet.org

BrainInjury.com
A medical, legal, and informational resource for persons dealing with traumatic brain injury
Web site: www.braininjury.com

Center for Disease Control (CDC)
National Center for Injury Prevention and Control site has a downloadable brochure *Facts about Concussion and Brain Injury and Where to Get Help*. This brochure explains what can happen after a concussion, how to get better, and where to go for more information and help when needed.
Web site: www.cdc.gov/ncipc/tbi

Centre for Neuro Skills (CNS)-TBI Resource Guide
The TBI Resource Guide from CNS is a main source of infor-

mation, services and products relating to TBI, BI recovery and post-acute rehabilitation. New on the Web site are an online drugstore and a virtual tour of the CNS brain injury rehab facilities. Web site features "Inside View" online newsletter and book of the week.

Web site: www.neuroskills.com

Craig Hospital Brain Injury Education Information

Web site: www.craighospital.org/TBI/healthAndWellness.asp

Defense and Veterans Brain Injury Center

The mission of the Defense and Veterans Brain Injury Center (DVBIC) is to serve active-duty military, their dependents, and veterans with TBI through state-of-the-art medical care, innovative clinical research initiatives, and educational programs.

1-800-870-9244 (DSN) 662-6345

E-mail: info@dvbic.org

Web site: www.dvbic.org

Head Injury Hotline

This is a nonprofit clearinghouse of information started in 1985 by survivors of brain injury. This resource provides a list of brain injury rehab facilities, understanding brain injury, a rehab checklist, a lawyer checklist, advocacy, goal setting, problem solving, library, chat, and TBI services and support groups.

Web site: www.headinjury.com

National Institute of Neurological Disorders and Stroke (NINDS) Traumatic Brain Injury Page

Web site: www.ninds.nih.gov/disorders/tbi/tbi.htm

National Resource Center for Traumatic Brain Injury
Traumatic brain injury Web site produced by the Virginia Commonwealth University/Medical College of Virginia. Includes guides for survivors; families, friends, and caregivers; living and working productively; and rehabilitation providers. Also provides TBI frequently asked questions (FAQs), chats with Pat, and directory of experts.

Web site: www.neuro.pmr.vcu.edu

NeuroSurgeryToday.org
Information site about TBI as well as other neurological conditions

Web site: www.neurosurgerytoday.org

The Perspectives Network (TPN)
This international nonprofit organization was founded in 1990 by a survivor of acquired brain injury. TPN offers a monthly publication and on-line resource information and support dealing with the consequences of traumatic brain injury.

E-mail: TPN@tbi.org

Web site: www.tbi.org

The Rehabilitation Research Center for TBI & SCI
Web site for the Rehabilitation Research Center at Santa Clara Valley Medical Center. Links to the TBIRD, the revised (November 2005) Traumatic Brain Injury Resource Directory (TBIRD), which lists hundreds of TBI-related resources in its 25 chapters. The TBIRD is available in print (for a fee) and on-line (for free!) at its TBIRD link: www.tbi-sci/tbird

Web site: www.tbi-sci.org

TraumaticBrainInjury.com

TraumaticBrainInjury is a project of TraumaticBrainInjury.
com, LLC. Our mission is to be the leading internet resource
for education, advocacy, research and support for brain injury
survivors, their families, and medical and rehabilitation professionals.

Web site: www.traumaticbraininjury.com

Traumatic Brain Injury Survival Guide

Online TBI survival guide book written by Glen Johnson,
Ph.D., clinical neuropsychologist from Michigan. Easy-to-read
chapters for the layperson include common indicators of head
injury, understanding how the brain works, coping with common problems, dealing with doctors, emotional stages of recov-
ers, returning to school, when will I get better, and who are all
those professionals.

Web site: www.tbiguide.com

Accessible Travel

Provided by MossRehab ResourceNet, this is an information
service for the traveler with a disability. They offer general help
as you make your travel plans. On this Web site are travel tips;
travel agencies; information on airlines, trains, and buses; ho-
tels/motels; van and car rental companies; government resources; newsgroups; and mailing lists.

Web site: www.mossresourcenet.org/travel.htm

Advocacy Groups

Mothers Against Drunk Driving (MADD)

MADD works to prevent the tragedy of drunk driving and prevent underage drinking. They are also committed to serving drunk driving victims and survivors.

24 Helpline: 1-877-MADD-HELP 1-877-623-3435
Web site: www.madd.org

National Domestic Violence Hotline

Information and advice about domestic violence; referrals to local resources and shelters.

Phone: 1-800-799-SAFE(7233) TTY: 1-800-787-3224
Web site: www.ndvh.org

Assistive Technology

AbilityHub

Assistive technology for people with a disability who find operating a computer difficult, maybe even impossible. This Web site will direct you to adaptive equipment and alternative methods available for accessing computers.

Web site: www.abilityhub.com

ABLEDATA

ABLEDATA provides objective information on assistive technology and rehabilitation equipment available from domestic and international sources to consumers, organizations, professionals, and caregivers within the United States. They serve the nation's disability, rehabilitation, and senior communities.

ABLEDATA is sponsored by the National Institute on Disability and Rehabilitation Research (NIDRR), part of the Office of Special Education and Rehabilitative Services (OSERS) of the U.S. Department of Education. They do not produce, distribute, or sell any of the products listed on the database, but provide you with information on how to contact manufacturers or distributors of these products.

Web site: www.abledata.com/

Brain Tumors

American Brain Tumor Association
The American Brain Tumor Association exists to eliminate brain tumors through research and to meet the needs of brain tumor patients and their families.

Web site: www.abta.org

The Brain Tumor Society
Web site contains information for the entire brain tumor community, from newly diagnosed patients to survivors, families, and healthcare professionals.

Web site: www.tbts.org

National Brain Tumor Foundation
The National Brain Tumor Foundation (NBTF) is a nationwide nonprofit organization serving people whose lives are affected by brain tumors. We are dedicated to promoting a cure for brain tumors, improving the quality of life, and giving hope to the brain tumor community by funding meaningful research and providing patient resources, timely information, and education.

Call for support 800-934-CURE

Web site: www.braintumor.org

Caregiver Support

Family Caregiver Alliance (FCA)
Assists families of persons with chronic or progressive brain disorders. Distributes information on caregiving and care of people with cognitive impairments. Web site contains fact sheets, articles, and links to state-level resources. Online interactive services include a support group for caregivers, problem-solving consultation, and "Ask FCA."

180 Montgomery Street, Suite 1100

San Francisco, CA 94104

Phone: 415-434-3388 (V); 800/445-8106

Fax: 415-434-3508

E-mail: info@caregiver.org

Web site: /www.caregiver.org

The TBI Help Desk for Caregivers

Mission: To enhance, expand and extend the quality of care available to caregivers and survivors of traumatic brain injury.

Web site: www.tbihelp.org

Community Integration

Information on life after TBI provided by the Rehabilitation Research and Training Center (RRTC) on community integration of persons with traumatic brain injury.

Web site: www.tbicommunity.org

Disability Information, Advocacy, Rights

ADA Home Page (U.S. Department of Justice)
Information and technical assistance with the Americans with Disabilities Act.

Web site: www.usdoj.gov/crt/ada/adahom1.htm

American Association of People with Disabilities
Web site: www.AAPD.com

ADA Technical Assistance Program and Regional Disability and Business Technical Assistance Centers
The National Institute on Disability and Rehabilitation Research has established a network of 10 regional Disability and Business Technical Assistance Centers. The DBTACs form a comprehensive national network for the provision of information and referrals, technical assistance, public awareness, and training on all aspects of the American with Disabilities Act.

Phone: 800-949-4232

Web site: www.adata.org

American Association of People with Disabilities
The AAPD is the largest national nonprofit cross-disability member organization in the United States, dedicated to ensuring economic self-sufficiency and political empowerment for the more than 56 million Americans with disabilities. The AAPD works in coalition with other disability organizations for the full implementation and enforcement of disability nondiscrimination laws, particularly the Americans with Disabilities Act of 1990 and the Rehabilitation Act of 1973.

Web site: www.aapd-dc.org

Americans with Disabilities Act

This information service answers questions on requirements set forth by the Americans with Disabilities Act and offers referrals to other government agencies involved with disability issues.

ADA Information Line: 202-514-0301

ADA Home Page: www.ada.gov

DisabilityInfo.gov

This site provides access to government-sponsored disability-related information and programs on numerous subjects, including civil rights, community life, education, employment, housing, health, income support, technology, and transportation. The site is the result of the New Freedom Initiative, which directed federal agencies to build a one-stop interagency portal for people with disabilities, their families, employers, service providers, and community members.

Web site: www.disabilityinfo.gov

Internet Resources for Special Children

The IRSC Web site is dedicated to children with disabilities and other health-related disorders worldwide.

Contains resource information and online communities for information and support.

Web site: www.irsc.org

National Council on Disability

The NCD's overall purpose is to promote policies, programs, practices, and procedures that guarantee equal opportunity for all individuals with disabilities, regardless of the nature or severity of the disability; and to empower individuals with disabilities to achieve economic self-sufficiency, independent living, and inclusion and integration into all aspects of society.

Web site: www.ncd.gov

National Disability Rights Network

Voluntary association of protection and advocacy systems and client-assistance programs. Promotes rigorous enforcement of laws protecting the civil and human rights of persons with disabilities, including those with TBI. Phone: 202-408-9514, 202-408-9521 (TTY)

Web site: www.ndrn.org

National Dissemination Center for Children with Disabilities

This is a central source of information on disabilities in infants, toddlers, children, and youth;

IDEA, which is the law authorizing special education; No Child Left Behind (as it relates to children with disabilities); and research-based information on effective educational practices. The Web site is devoted to providing information on disabilities for families, educators, and other professionals. Special focus is on children and youth (birth to age 22). Services include personal responses to specific questions, publications, referrals to other disability organizations, and information searches for their own library and databases. Information is also provided in Spanish.

Web site: www.nichcy.org

World Association of Persons with Disabilities

The WAPD advances the interests of persons with disabilities at national, state, local, and home levels. We believe that all are entitled to high quality of life

Web site: www.wapd.org

Education

Educating Educators About ABI
Web site: www.abieducation.com

Lash and Associates Publishing/Training
Publisher committed to helping families, survivors, clinicians, teachers, advocates, and counselors recognize and respond to the special needs of children, adolescents, and young adults with brain injuries and other disabilities. Information and training on brain injury in adults and youths for educators, clinicians, therapists, parents, and survivors.

Web site: www.lapublishing.com/

General Health Information

American Speech-Language, Hearing Association
This nonprofit organization provides educational information on speech, language, and hearing disabilities. The association publishes pamphlets and other literature on a wide range of communication disorders. It also provides referrals for speech and language pathologists in specific localities.

10801 Rockville Pike
Rockville, MD 20852
Telephone: 800-498-2071 or 301-897-8682
TTY: 301-897-8682
Web site: www.asha.org

Centers for Disease Control (use Search for specific information)
Web site: www.cdc.gov

Healthfinder
Guide to reliable health information, sponsored by the Office of Disease Prevention and Health Promotion, U.S. Department of Health and Human Services.
Web site: www.healthfinder.gov

Medscape
This site has the full text of articles from such sources as the National Institutes of Health and the Centers for Disease Control and Prevention.
Web site: www.medscape.com

National Institute on Deafness and Other Communication Disorders
Health information, including information on brain injury. Information is also available in Spanish
Web site: www.nidcd.nih.gov/health/voice/tbrain.asp

National Institutes of Health
Health Information
Web site: http://health.nih.gov/

National Institute of Neurological Disorders and Stroke
The mission of NINDS is to reduce the burden of neurological disease, a burden borne by every age group, by every segment of society, by people all over the world. This is done by supporting research and the dissemination of research information related to neurological disorders.
Web site: www.ninds.nih.gov

The National Library of Medicine
The National Library of Medicine provides two free systems to search medical topics in the MEDLINE database. About 11 million references and abstracts are found in this database.

Web site: www.ncbi.nih.gov/entrez/query.fcgi

NOAH (New York Online Access to Health)
NOAH provides access to high-quality consumer health information in English and Spanish. Librarians and health professionals in New York and beyond find, select, and organize full-text consumer health information that is current, relevant, accurate, and unbiased.

Web site: www.noah-health.org

Optometrists Network
Web site dedicated to eye therapy, with goal to help people find eye doctors who can help them. Site also provides useful patient education, free to the public, with no registration required.

Web site: www.vision3d.com

SafeUSA
Working to make our nation's homes, schools, worksites, transportation areas, and communities safer, SafeUSA is dedicated to eliminating unintentional and violent injury and death in America.

Web site: www.cdc.gov/safeusa

The Whole Brain Atlas
This is your brain in pictures, an incredible collection of magnetic resonance imaging (MRI) images of the brain.

Web site: www.med.harvard.edu/AANLIB/home.html

Independent Living

Independent Living Centers
Independent Living Centers are typically nonresidential, private, nonprofit, consumer-controlled, community-based organizations providing services and advocacy by and for persons with all types of disabilities. Their goal is to assist individuals with disabilities to achieve their maximum potential within their families and communities. Also, Independent Living Centers serve as a strong advocacy voice on a wide range of national, state, and local issues. They work to assure physical and programmatic access to housing, employment, transportation, communities, recreational facilities, and health and social services. These are just a few of the services offered. There are nearly 500 ILCs in the United States.

Directories by state:
www.virtualcil.net/cils
www.ilusa.com/links/ilcenters

National Council on Independent Living
As a membership organization, NCIL advances independent living and the rights of people with disabilities through consumer-driven advocacy. The NCIL envisions a world in which people with disabilities are valued equally and participate fully.

Web site: www.ncil.org

Legal Resources

Brain Injury Law Group
The Brain Injury Law Group is a community of plaintiff's trial lawyers across the United States, serving the rights of persons

with TBI. The Web site provides an 800 number to assist survivors of TBI in locating a lawyer specializing in brain injury in the state where they were injured. Also features articles, information, and graphics about TBI.

Web site: www.tbilaw.com

Neurolaw

Provides useful information about the incidence, causes, and consequences of brain injury (BI) and SCI, new developments in diagnosis and treatment, a glossary of BI and SCI terms, medico-legal issues affecting survivors and their families, and information about resources available to BI/SCI survivors and family members.

Web site: www.neurolaw.com

Mental Health

Mental Health Net

The mission of the Mental Help Net Web site is to promote mental health and wellness education and advocacy.

Web site: www.mhnet.org/

National Alliance for the Mentally Ill (NAMI)

NAMI is the nation's largest grassroots mental health organization dedicated to improving the lives of persons living with serious mental illness and their families. Founded in 1979, NAMI has become the nation's voice on mental illness, a national organization including NAMI organizations in every state and in over 1,100 local communities across the country who join together to meet the NAMI mission through advocacy, research, support, and education.

Web site: www.nami.org

National Institute of Mental Health

The National Institute of Mental Health (NIMH) is the largest scientific organization in the world dedicated to research focused on the understanding, treatment, and prevention of mental disorders and the promotion of mental health.

Web site: www.nimh.nih.gov

Quackery/Health Fraud

The National Council Against Health Fraud

A good place to get more information about questionable health claims and practices.

Web site: www.ncahf.org

Quackwatch, Inc.

A nonprofit corporation whose purpose is to combat health-related frauds, myths, fads, fallacies, and misconduct. Its primary focus is on quackery-related information that is difficult or impossible to get elsewhere. The Web site also *provides links to hundreds of reliable health sites.*

Web site: www.quackwatch.com

Rehabilitation

The National Rehabilitation Information Center

A site with an abundance of disability- and rehabilitation-oriented information organized in a variety of formats designed to make it easy for users to find and use. For the past 25 years, NARIC staff members have been dedicated to providing direct, personal, and high-quality information services to anyone through-out the country. As a leader in providing interactive information to the disability and rehabilitation community, NARIC's Web site continues this tradition by putting the information into the hands of the users through online publications, searchable data-bases, and timely reference and referral data.

There are multiple information request options available:

By Phone: 800-346-2742. An information specialist will answer your call. If no information specialists are available, you may leave a message, including your telephone number with area code, and an information specialist will return your call.

By Chat: Click the Ask! icon on any page to begin a live ses-sion with an information specialist. This service is only available during business hours. Off-hours, you may leave a message, and an information specialist will reply within one business day.

By E-mail: Information and document requests can be e-mailed to naricinfo@heitechservices.com Due to copyright re-strictions, they cannot send full documents via e-mail.

By Fax: Fax an information or document request to 301-459-4263. Please include your contact information.

By Mail: Send information and document requests to:
NARIC
8201 Corporate Drive, Suite 600,
Landover, MD 20785
Web site: www.naric.com

The Rehabilitation Research Center for TBI and Spinal Cord Injury Web

This site contains information on the activities of the RRC as well as a large collection of easily accessible online resources, including resource guides, educational materials, newsletters, and bulletin boards.

Web site: www.tbi-sci.org

TBI Chat Groups

TBI Home

A peer-support Web site for people living with brain injury, their families, and friends to support each other by sharing their experiences.

Web site: www.tbihome.org

BrainInjuryChat.org

Provides peer support for people living with brain injury. Their purpose is to provide people who are living with brain injury a safe place to meet for support and information.

www.braininjurychat.org

Safety

American Medical ID

Features custom-engraved medical identification bracelet and necklace styles. Important information on medical conditions, drug and food allergies, prescribed medicines, and emergency contacts can be engraved onto the surface of a medical identification jewelry piece. Medical IDs are recommended by physicians and healthcare organizations throughout the world. Wearing a medical ID offers you and your loved ones peace of mind.

Web site: http://americanmedical-id.com/

Brain Injury Books

Brainlash: Maximize Your Recovery from Mild Brain Injury, 3rd Edition by Gail L. Denton, PhD

The author is a retired psychotherapist and a brain injury survivor. The book proves the tools and facts to make recovery of brain injury more intelligible. It covers every aspect of the recovery process, from driving and sex to self-esteem, stamina, support systems, nutrition, pain, and more.

Web site: www.brainlash.com

Children with Traumatic Brain Injury: A Parent's Guide. Edited by Lisa Schoenbrodt, Ed. D.

This is a comprehensive, must-have reference that provides parents with the support and information they need to help their child recover from a closed-head injury and to prevent further incidents.

Coping with Mild Traumatic Brain Injury: A Guide to Living with Problems Associated with Brain Trauma by Diane Stoler

Dr. Diane Roberts Stoler, Ed.D., a health psychologist and professional speaker, sustained a stroke from a cerebral bleed and two traumatic brain injuries (an auto accident and brain surgery). This reference book applies to all aspects of brain trauma, including concussion, stroke, and brain tumor. It describes the most common physical, mental, and psychological symptoms of brain injury, explaining why each occurs and what can be done about it, as well as offering practical suggestions for coping with the problem. Also covered are financial, insurance, and family issues; the rehabilitation process; and eventual outcomes. An extensive resource section provides additional guidance and sources of support.

Web site: www.drdiane.com

Head Injury: Information and Answers to Commonly Asked Questions: A Family's Guide to Coping by Christopher D. Sturm, Thomas R. Forget, Janet L. Sturm

Provides general information and answers to commonly asked questions regarding the aspects of severe head injury. Topics include: the accident, types of head injury, symptoms and behavior, intensive-care setting, prognosis and outcomes, emotional reactions, aspects of therapy, prevention, and glossary of terms.

I'll Carry the Fork by Kara Swenson

Death didn't find Kara Swanson the day the minivan careened into her own car, but the head injury she sustained changed her life forever. Traumatic brain injury (TBI) is not a laughing matter, but the author presents her painful tale in an Erma Bombeck-like style that wraps the hard information in humor and gentle playfulness. Alongside Kara's inspirational sense of humor, medical and legal professionals offer technical input and practical advice to those dealing with or helping someone through the aftermath of brain injury. This funny and informative book will help countless others find their way to a new life, and know that they are not alone on the journey.

Living with Brain Injury: A Guide for Families by Richard Senelick, M.D. and Karla Dougherty.

The new, updated edition of the renowned classic—complete with cutting-edge neuroplasticity and exciting experimental rehabilitation research! *Living with Brain Injury* will help readers, both families of patients and professionals alike, through new, uncharted territory of brain rehabilitation, a world where people we love may change before our eyes, physically, mentally, and emotionally.

Over My Head: A Doctor's Own Story of Head Injury from the Inside Looking Out by Claudia L. Osborn

Locked inside a brain-injured head looking out at a challenging world is the premise of this extraordinary autobiography. *Over My Head* is an inspiring story of how one woman comes to terms with the loss of her identity and the courageous steps (and hilarious missteps) she takes while learning to rebuild her life. The author, a 45-year-old doctor and clinical professor of medicine, describes the aftermath of a brain injury 11 years ago, which stripped her of her beloved profession. For years, she was deprived of her intellectual companionship and the ability to handle the simplest undertakings like shopping for groceries or sorting the mail. Her progression from confusion, dysfunction, and alienation to a full, happy life is told with restraint, great style, and considerable humor.

Web site: www.claudiaosborn.com

Traumatic Head Injury: Cause, Consequence and Challenge by Dennis P. Swiercinsky, Terrie L. Price, and Lief Erick Leaf

This book is a guide for understanding the causes and consequences of head injury, and the rehabilitation challenge for regaining as much functional independence as possible for adjusting to that which cannot be changed.

Local and State Resources

State Division of Vocational Rehabilitation
State agency that provides vocational rehabilitation services individuals with disabilities. Services can include counseling, advocacy, job training, job placements, and a variety of additional support services including continuing, adult, and postsecondary education. For the Office of Vocational Rehabilitation Services in your State, consult a phone directory or search online.

Rehabilitation agencies and hospitals: Contact local rehabilitation center departments for outpatient support programs

Local park and recreation agencies may have programs for special groups, including those with disabilities or more specifically, those with brain injuries.

Tools

Chapter 1: Put Your House In Order

Diet

American Dietetic Association
216 W. Jackson Boulevard
Chicago, IL 60606-6995
800-366-1655 (recorded messages)
900-225-5267 (to talk to a registered dietitian)
Web site: www.eatright.org

Nutrition and Your Health: Dietary Guidelines for Americans
Web site: http://198.102.218.57/dietaryguidelines/dga2000/document/frontcover.htm

U.S. Department of Agricultures MyPyramid.gov
Web site offers food patterns are designed for the general public ages 2 and over. They are not therapeutic diets for specific health conditions. MyPyramid Plan offers you a personal eating plan with the foods and amounts that are right for you. MyPyramid Tracker offers a detailed assessment of your food intake and physical activity level. Advice offered is based on your pyramid to help you make smart choices from every food group, and to find your balance between food and physical activity, get the most nutrition out of your calories, and stay within your daily calorie needs.
Web site: MyPyramid.gov

Supplements
FDA, Center for Food Safety and Applied Nutrition
Web site: www.cfsan.fda.gov/~dms/supplmnt.html

Exercise
American College of Sports Medicine Exercise Guidelines
Web site: www.acsm.org/health+fitness/index.htm
American Heart Association
Start! is the American Heart Association's groundbreaking national campaign that calls on all Americans and their employers to create a culture of physical fitness.
Web site: www.americanheart.org/start

Centers for Disease Control and Prevention Physical Activity Recommendations

Web site: www.cdc.gov/nccdphp/dnpa/physical/recommendations/index.htm

The President's Council on Physical Fitness and Sports

Web site: www.fitness.gov/fitness.htm

Stress Reduction

FamilyDoctor.org

Stress: How to Cope Better With Life's Challenges

Web site: www.familydoctor.org/167.xml

Mountain State Centers for Independent Living

Understanding and Dealing with Stress

Web site: www.mtstcil.org/skills/stress-intro.html

WebMD: Stress Management Health Center

Web site: www.Webmd.com/balance/stress-management/stress-management-topic-overview

Chapter 4: Checklists and Routines

Financial Software

Search online for sites that compare features of financial software to find the one that fits your needs best.

Microsoft Money

Web site: www.microsoft.com/money/

Quicken

Web site: www.quicken.com

Chapter 5: Attention

Ear Filters

Customized hearing protection that filters out background noise, the ER-9, ER-15, ER-25. Ask for this product at a hearing aid store or consult an audiologist.

To replace filters: http://earplugstore.stores.yahoo.net/er915and25pr.html

Ear plugs can be found at building supply/hardware stores, hardware departments in general merchandise stores.

Chapter 6: Memory

Back Packs

Back packs can be found at general merchandise and sporting goods stores as well as online at specialty retail stores. I have found ones to fit my needs at LL Bean: www.llbean.com, REI: www.REI.com, Sierra Trading Post: www.sierratradingpost.com and Campmor: www.campmor.com.

Carabiners

Carabiners can be found in the lock/key section of hardware or building supply stores, camping section of sporting goods, and in general merchandise stores.

Digital Recorder

Digital recorders can be found in office supply, electronics, and general merchandise stores as well as online. Some can be connected to your computer and download files. The files can then be listened to on the computer as well as stored.

Label Printers

Handheld:

Brother. Link to adviser to help chose desired features: www.advizia.com/brother/Advisor.asp?User=ptouch&Rnd=809

Dymo. http://global.dymo.com/enUS/Categories/Handheld_Labelmakers.html

There are also labels that can be printed either with your regular computer printer or a dedicated label printer. Printers are available at office supply and electronics stores as well as online.

Pill Management Systems

Simple daily/weekly/monthly pill containers are available in most pharmacies/pharmacy sections of general merchandise stores.

Talking or alarm pill reminder systems are available. Many can be found online, or you can check with your pharmacist for suggestions.

B Independent solutions, from the Net's only store created by and for brain injury survivors and families, has multiple systems available. </bl>
Web site: www.bindependent.com/

Personal Digital Assistants (PDAs)
You can search online for comparisons of currently available PDAs. PC World (www.pcworld.com) and PC Magazine (www.pcmag.com) are two locations where you can find helpful information. It is very helpful to go to a store carrying multiple brands and have the salesperson show you the different features and how to operate them. Ask around for friends and family

who use PDAs to get recommendations and help in selecting and using a PDA.

PDAs can be bought online, at office supply or electronics stores, and at large general merchandise and warehouse stores.

Schedulers/Planners
Simple to complex, inexpensive to expensive:
Office Supply Stores or office supply departments in general merchandise stores
Franklin Day Planner:
800-654-1776
www.franklincovey.com

Day-Timer:
800-225-5005
www.daytimer.com

Sticky Notes
Sticky notes can be found in office supply stores as well as the school supply sections of general merchandise stores.
Freeware Computer Stickies
Web site: www.zhornsoftware.co.uk

Chapter 7: Time Management

Alarms and Timers
B Independent solutions, from the Net's only store created by and for brain injury survivors and families has multiple alarm and timer options.
Web site: www.bindependent.com/

Portable Timers

Portable timers can be found in the kitchen goods departments in general merchandise stores.

Wall Calendars, Blackboards, Dry-erase Board Organizational Systems

I have found organizational systems I like at Pottery Barn

Web site: www.potterybarn.com Look under Accessories, Storage and Organization

Office supply stores, office supply section of general merchandise stores

Watches

Watches with one to three daily alarms are generally available at jewelry, sporting goods, and general merchandise stores. Watches with more alarms, or vibrating functions are also available and many options can be found with online searches or at B Independent, Web site: www.bindependent.com/

Chapter 9: Communication

Software to deal with speech, language recovery after stroke or other type of brain injury

Web site: www.bungalowsoftware.com

Chapter 10: Transportation

Mapping Programs for Driving

Google

Mapquest-www.mapquest.com

Yahoo

Miscellaneous

Fun and Games/Brain Exercises

AARP Games

Features free online puzzles, jigsaws, and other interactive games. The site includes clear instructions with few advertising interruptions.

Web site: www.aarpmagazine.org/games/

Pogo.com

Offers free games such as whomp, solitaire, dominoes, chess, and more. Registration is required to play games on this site. It is quick, easy, and worthwhile to register because of the wide variety of games.

Web site: www.pogo.com/home/home.jsp?sls=2&site =pogo

All Games Free

Offers a wide variety of free games including arcade games, card games, puzzle and word games, sports games, and interactive trivia games. Registration is fast and free and, once you're registered, you will be able to create a custom "my games page," with all of your favorite games.

Web site: www.allgamesfree.com/

Free Arcade

Features more than 150 arcade games such as puzzle games, board games, and card games without required logins or sign ups.

Web site: www.freearcade.com/

PopCap Games

A commercial site featuring both single-player and networked games. The single-player games include fun, speed-based games like Big Money and Diamond Mine as well as puzzle solvers like Atomica and Mummy Maze. To play, click on a game; it will take a few minutes to load.

Web site: www.popcap.com/

Playsite

Offers networked gaming; you can play games with people from all over the world. Choices include board games (Monopoly, chess, backgammon, and more), card games (bridge, hearts, spades, euchre, and more), word games (Scrabble, Tangleword), classic arcade games (Asteroids, Centipede), and more. Registration is required.

Web site: www.iwin.com/

Play Free Online Games

Offers a great selection of free games, including adventure games, arcade games, board games, cards, sports, puzzles, word games, etc. Some you will need to sign up for, others just click and play.

Web site: www.playfreeonlinegames.co.uk/

MSN Games

Provides a good selection of board and card games that are especially easy to access and play. Provides helpful hints for the games, if needed, and features good game descriptions and the ability to browse by genre.

Web site: http://zone.msn.com/en/root/default.htm

Zeeks! Games

Offers all sorts of games, with few advertisers. Some games may be appropriate to play with your children and grandchildren.

Web site: http://games.zeeks.com/games.php

Merriam-Webster Online

A commercial site, offering a new word game every day. Features four types of games based on words, definitions, and etymology. Includes an archive of two months of games. To play, click on "play today's word game" and wait a few moments for the game to load.

Web site: www.merriam-Webster.com/game/

Cartoon Network

Network (commercial) site that includes free games.

Web site: www.cartoonnetwork.com/games/index.html

Online Jigsaw Puzzles

Some sites include capability to determine difficulty level of puzzle, be timed doing a puzzle and compare to others, and have daily puzzle e-mailed to you.

www.castlib.dk/free-online-jigsaw-puzzle-and-puzzle-games.php

www.freejigsawpuzzles.com/

www.liessmit.nl/html/puzzles.htm

www.jigsawplanet.com/

www.jigzone.com/

Either I could be bad at trying to be the person I'd been before I got sick, or I could figure out who I was now and learn to be good at that.

Edward Readicker-Henderson

Index

My Story

I wanted to be a doctor since I was young. After four years of college, four years of medical school, and three years of a Family Medicine residency, I was finally free to live out my dream. I first spent two years in the rural thumb area of Michigan, paying back the National Health Service Corps for financial help with my schooling. I then practiced for eight years in a mostly solo family practice in Mt. Pleasant Michigan before deciding that the office part of the practice of medicine, the personal interaction with patients and teaching them how to stay healthy and out of hospitals, was what I loved the most. I moved to Colorado to work for Kaiser Permanente, a non-profit HMO, where I could do office-based medicine and where I was encouraged to continue my love of community education. I moved into a part time management position, with still most of my time spent in direct patient care. I would have been happy doing this all of my life, but that was not to happen.

In February of 2002 a friend loaned me her log cabin in the mountains for a relaxing weekend getaway. I was able to ski at Winter Park as well as snowshoe and cross-country ski near her cabin, just outside of the Rocky Mountain National Park. I had a wonderful weekend; restful time spent recharging my emotional batteries. On my way home I decided to get in a couple of last runs on the ski slope, enjoying a few inches of new powder on the ground. On my first run I stopped for a sight seeing break and somehow slipped and fell backwards, hitting my helmeted head on ice under the few inches of powder. I thought I'd just "rung my bell," but as I was later to learn, that concussion on top of multiple previous ones started a new chapter in my life.

After my 2002 traumatic brain injury (TBI), I was continuing to have difficulty dealing with the losses I'd had, both in my own self's functioning abilities and the related loss of my career. In 2005 I had a near-fatal car accident, with resultant injuries that were potentially life threatening. As I recovered from these injuries, my father had a near-fatal fall, fracturing his neck and, as we later learned, sustaining a TBI. Almost the entire year was wiped out in dealing with these issues. Just as I was getting my feet under me in 2006, with my 12-year-old Boston terrier at risk for dying due to a faulty heart valve, my younger, healthy Boston terrier developed a brain tumor. Fortunately, it was a type sensitive to radiation treatment and he responded well. When I asked his vet what might be the consequences of the tumor and treatment in relationship to his cognitive function, I was told "he only has to be a dog." This concept caught my attention, as he would likely be as happy as before, even with cognitive changes, as he didn't expect himself to be a perfectly performing dog.

I began 2007 with a new attitude, that being a doctor was what I did, not who I was. I also came to realize that in the scope of life, being alive and in pretty good physical condition as well as having the ability and means to take care of myself was a pretty good thing. I also finally realized that in life, the journey is as important as the destination. I decided to travel, visiting the last of the 50 states I'd yet to visit, and while traveling resumed work on the Brain Injury Tools book I'd started before my car accident and had set aside.

My 2007 journey eventually led me to visit all of the 50 states in my 50th year and to meet many extraordinary people along the journey, many with personal or family experience with brain injury. The book I'd labored to start two years previously seemed to just write itself. 2007 was the year I finally found peace and was able to accept the new me and leave behind my medical career and the person I had been before my accident. I came to realize that I am where I'm supposed to be. I now know that with my background in medicine, medical administration, and community education as well as my personal and family experience with brain injury, I can be a resource to others.

I hope as I continue my journey I can help others dealing with brain injury to better understand and deal with the changes in themselves, their family members or their friends. I also hope to help remove the title "Silent Epidemic" from brain injury by speaking publicly wherever and whenever possible in order to raise the knowledge and understanding of this topic among the medical and general public. Let the journey begin!

Special discounts on bulk quantities of Demos Medical Publishing books are available to corporations, professional associations, pharmaceutical companies, health care organizations, and other qualifying groups. For details, please contact:
Special Sales Department
Demos Medical Publishing
11 W. 42nd St., 15th Floor
New York, NY 10036
Phone: 800–532–8663 or 212–683–0072
Fax: 212–683–0118
E-mail: orderdept@demosmedpub.com

Library of Congress Cataloging-in-Publication Data
Sullivan, Cheryle.
  Brain injury survival kit : 365 tips, tools & tricks to deals with cognitive function loss / Cheryle Sullivan.
    p. cm.
  Includes index.
  ISBN-13: 978-1-932603-73-6 (pbk. : alk. paper)
  ISBN-10: 1-932603-73-5 (pbk. : alk. paper)
  1. Brain damage—Popular works. I. Title.
  RC387.5.S85 2009
  617.4'81044—dc22

                                                                2008017420

11 12   9 8 7 6 5

Brain Injury Survival Kit

365 Tips, Tools, & Tricks to Deal with
Cognitive Function Loss

Cheryle Sullivan, MD

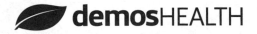

demosHEALTH